AF521616

MEDICAL HISTORY AND MEDICAL CARE

MEDICAL HISTORY AND MEDICAL CARE

A symposium of perspectives

Arranged by the Nuffield Provincial Hospitals Trust
and the Josiah Macy Jr Foundation

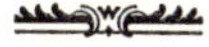

CONTRIBUTORS
THOMAS McKEOWN, GEORGE ROSEN
JOHN BROTHERSTON, PAUL SANAZARO
BERNARD TOWERS, RASHI FEIN
HENRY MILLER AND JOHN BOWERS

WITH A PREFACE BY
LORD COHEN OF BIRKENHEAD

EDITED BY GORDON McLACHLAN
AND THOMAS McKEOWN

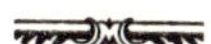

Published for the Nuffield Provincial Hospitals Trust
by the Oxford University Press
London New York Toronto
1971

Oxford University Press, Ely House, London W1

GLASGOW NEW YORK TORONTO MELBOURNE WELLINGTON
CAPE TOWN SALISBURY IBADAN NAIROBI DAR ES SALAAM LUSAKA ADDIS ABABA
BOMBAY CALCUTTA MADRAS KARACHI LAHORE DACCA
KUALA LUMPUR SINGAPORE HONG KONG TOKYO

ISBN 0 19 721362 6

Designed by Bernard Crossland

PRINTED IN GREAT BRITAIN
BY HAZELL WATSON AND VINEY LTD
AYLESBURY, BUCKS

It is impossible to understand the present without knowing the past

GOETHE

Contents

Preface

LORD COHEN OF BIRKENHEAD

On 20th and 21st October 1970, a symposium on 'Medical History and Medical Care' was held in London under the joint auspices of the Nuffield Provincial Hospitals Trust and the Josiah Macy Jr Foundation. It aimed to explore and evaluate the history of the human experience of disease—its prevention, cure, and alleviation; the genetic and environmental factors which have determined its incidence in different ages and in varying social and political climates; the medical care which populations have received through diverse channels, their social attitudes to such care, and its effects on the health of the people.

The aim had, of course, a goal which was to ascertain how far such historical studies help to provide a fruitful perspective, capable of contributing to the solution of contemporary problems. 'The farther you look back,' observed Sir Winston Churchill, 'the farther forward you can see.'

Yet it cannot be denied that many distinguished historians deny a 'pragmatic' history (to use Polybius' term) which, by example from times past, provides a guide to the interpretation and elucidation of present problems.

The eight papers and the summary of the discussion presented at the symposium which are included in this volume, will, we trust, help the reader to decide for himself whether this historical approach to the problems of social or community medicine has proved profitable.

The papers as printed here are revised versions of those

presented to the symposium. This enabled each participant, if he thought fit, to refine his own approach and judgement after hearing and assessing the views of his fellows. A bare recital of the topics discussed reflects the nature of our inquiry. These included the unmasking of the means of controlling disease at different epochs, and of promoting health; the evolution of diverse systems of medical care especially in the United Kingdom and United States of America; the relative roles of institutional and domiciliary care; the control of population growth, and the care of the mentally sick, the aged, and disabled; the administrative structure of health services; priorities in medical care; and cost/benefit problems which arise in the economics of medical care and in the increasing use and complexity of modern techniques in diagnosis and treatment. What effect should the rapidly expanding corpus of medical knowledge have on the training of those responsible for the provision of medical care? How far is the general public aware of the benefits of medical care and prepared to exert political pressure to ensure its availability to those in need; and so forth?

One of the most striking features of this exercise was the increasing recognition during its course that none of these facets of medical care can exist in isolation. Each represents a thread whose course continues with all others to create a tapestry of recognizable design.

It is far too early to assess the ultimate value of this symposium. Perhaps as much was gained in the informal meetings with one's colleagues as in the more formal sessions, and perhaps future meetings of similar type will help to illuminate the persisting shadows. But few who were privileged to take part in these two intensive days of study and discussion will doubt the truth of Santayana's dictum that those who neglect the study of history are compelled to relive it.

No symposium such as this can take place without an enormous amount of planning editorially. Special thanks are due to Dr John Z. Bowers, Professor Thomas McKeown, and Mr Gordon McLachlan, who were responsible for its shape and direction.

Liverpool, March 1971

List of participants

PAUL BEESON, MD, FRCP, Nuffield Professor of Clinical Medicine, University of Oxford.

GEORGE PACKER BERRY, MD, Member of Board of Directors, Josiah Macy Jr Foundation, New York.

JOHN Z. BOWERS, MD, President, Josiah Macy Jr Foundation, New York.

JOHN BROTHERSTON, MA, MD, FRCP, DPH, Chief Medical Officer, Scottish Home and Health Department, Edinburgh.

EDWIN CLARKE, MD, MRCP, Senior Lecturer in History of Medicine, University College, London.

LORD COHEN OF BIRKENHEAD, DSC, MD, FRCP, HON FRCS, LLD, FSA, DCL, DL, JP,[1, 2] President, General Medical Council.

RASHI FEIN, PHD, Professor of the Economics of Medicine, Harvard University Medical School, Boston.

JOHN FRY, MD, FRCS, FRCGP,[1] General Practitioner, London.

ROBERT J. GLASER, MD, Vice-President, The Commonwealth Fund, New York.

JOHN R. HOGNESS, MD, Director of Health Sciences Center, University of Washington, Seattle.

E. HUGH LUCKEY, MD, President, The New York Hospital, Cornell Medical Center, New York.

THOMAS MCKEOWN, PHD, DPHIL, MD, FRCP, Professor of Social Medicine, University of Birmingham.

GORDON MCLACHLAN, CBE, BCOM, FCA,[3] Secretary, Nuffield Provincial Hospitals Trust, London.

HENRY MILLER, MD, FRCP, DPM, Vice-Chancellor, University of Newcastle upon Tyne.

S. G. OWEN, MD, FRCP, Second Secretary, Medical Research Council, London.

OSLER L. PETERSON, MD, Professor of Preventive Medicine, Harvard University Medical School, Boston.

SIR GEORGE PICKERING, DSc, MA, FRCP, FRS, Master of Pembroke College, University of Oxford.

H. N. ROBSON, FRCP, FRACP,[1] Vice-Chancellor, University of Sheffield.

GEORGE ROSEN, MD, Professor of the History of Medicine and Epidemiology and Public Health, Yale University School of Medicine, New Haven.

LORD ROSENHEIM, KBE, MA, MD, PRCP, President of the Royal College of Physicians of London and Professor of Medicine, University of London.

PAUL J. SANAZARO, MD, Director, National Center for Health Services Research and Development, Washington.

BERNARD TOWERS, MA, MB, CHB, Professor of Paediatrics and Anatomy, The University of California, Los Angeles.

E. T. WILLIAMS, CB, CBE, DSO, DL,[1, 4] Warden of Rhodes House, Oxford.

HENRY YELLOWLEES, CB, MRCP, Deputy Chief Medical Officer, Department of Health and Social Security, London.

1. Governing trustee of the Nuffield Provincial Hospitals Trust.
2. Chairman of Symposium. 3. Secretary of Symposium.
4. Chairman of the Nuffield Provincial Hospitals Trust.

I

A SOCIOLOGICAL APPROACH TO THE HISTORY OF MEDICINE

THOMAS McKEOWN

A sociological approach to the history of medicine[1]

What history can teach is a much discussed question and historians themselves are divided about the answer; what medical history can teach is a question which is not often asked and yet there can be little doubt about the answer. The direction of medical effort, both in service and research, is seriously prejudiced because of lack of the perspective which historical investigation could provide.

The provision of this perspective, I suggest, should be the main aim of the social historian and I have taken my title from Sigerist's essay on *The Social History of Medicine* in which he wrote:

> I would like to draw your attention to a field of studies in the history of medicine that has been greatly neglected in the past. If you open a textbook, any textbook of medical history, and try to find what health conditions were in rural France in the eighteenth century, or what disease meant to the family of an artisan at the same period, you will as a rule not find any information. We know much about the great medical discoveries but very little on whether they were applied or to whom they were applied.

Sigerist ended his essay with these words: 'I think that the sociological approach to the history of medicine not only gives us a better understanding of the past but can also help us in

1. This paper is a modified version of the Inaugural Lecture of the Society for the Social History of Medicine. It is published with the permission of the Society and of *Medical History*, in which it was originally published (*Medical History*, vol. iv, no. 4 [October 1970]).

planning the future.' On this interpretation, if social history is history with the politics left out, the social history of medicine is medical history with the public interest put in.

It is not difficult to suggest why this interest has hitherto been lacking. Those who have taken up the study of medical history have done so mainly for love of history; being fascinated by the lives and work of men such as Hippocrates, Galen, and Osler, they seem scarcely to have noticed that these giants were unable to treat any disease effectively. In consequence, histories of medicine, like histories of art, have two main themes, the great men and the great movements. Leonardo and the High Renaissance; Pasteur and the rise of bacteriology. A case could be made for the view that the best statistician is the one who dislikes figures and the safest surgeon the one who does not enjoy operating; perhaps the most successful social historian would be one who does not particularly care for history, but turns to it because he considers it indispensable to an understanding of contemporary problems. From this viewpoint the social history of medicine is much more than a blend of social history and medical history, more than medical developments seen in the social context of their period; it is essentially an operational approach which takes its terms of reference from difficulties confronting medicine in the present day. It is the lack of such insight, derived from contemporary experience, which makes a good deal of medical history so sterile for the uninitiated.

I shall devote the remainder of this paper to discussion of some problems which illustrate the scope of the work which awaits the attention of the social historian.

1. INFLUENCES ON MAN'S HEALTH

Since the seventeenth century it has been thought that improvements in health must be based on an understanding of the structure and function of the body and the disease processes which affect it. This concept has been largely responsible for the significance attached to the work of the acute hospital and for the relative neglect of psychiatric, geriatric, and some other forms of care; it has had a powerful influence on the direction of medical research. If the concept remains unchallenged, it is probable that these trends will be exaggerated in future and that medicine will become still more sharply divided into favoured and depressed areas, based on a division between technology and care.

It is therefore imperative that there should be a critical evaluation of the influences on which human health depends. Such an investigation must be largely historical, an examination of the conditions under which man developed and of the major influences which affected health at different stages of his evolution. I believe the conclusions will lead to a picture very different from the one which has been predominant since the seventeenth century.

2. WHAT DOCTORS HAVE BEEN DOING

Non-medical writers have not hesitated to make their own evaluation of the medical measures of their day and some have arrived at low estimates. The views of Montaigne and Shaw, for example, are particularly explicit; those of Tolstoy in *War and Peace* include a characteristically profound appraisal of the medical task as well as a judgement on the ineffectiveness of treatment.

In spite of the literary distinction of the critics such opinions have been largely ignored by medical people, or regarded as so perverse that they do not merit serious consideration. Historians in particular have shown little interest in assessment of the character of doctors' work and the extent of their achievement at different periods in history; in general they have been interested in what was done rather than in whether it was worth doing.

As a background to present and future developments in medicine it seems essential to put the work and achievement of the past into much clearer perspective. The following analysis suggests the lines such an inquiry might take and a few tentative conclusions derived from it.

The tasks on which doctors have been traditionally engaged may be classified as follows:

a. Diagnosis or identification of disease

Although several diseases were recognized with more or less certainty at an earlier date (for example, smallpox, plague, dysentery, tetanus, rabies, gonorrhoea, and syphilis) reliable identification of disease began in the nineteenth century.

b. Pathology or understanding of disease

In spite of earlier advances in related sciences such as anatomy and physiology, an accurate understanding of disease processes was delayed until the ninetenth century. It owed much to recognition of the bacterial origin of infections.

c. Prevention of disease

Although some reforms were anticipated earlier, effective preventive measures began with the control of the environment in the second half of the nineteenth century. Vaccination against smallpox was the only means of preventing disease in the individual before 1900.

d. Cure of disease

Effective treatment began in the twentieth century. Some useful drugs were introduced much earlier (for example, mercury, iron, quinine, and digitalis) but the circumstances and manner of their use, and the limited grasp of their mode of action suggest that they must have been relatively ineffective. Before the discovery of anaesthesia, operations were mainly for cataracts, amputations, incisions for abscesses, lithotomy, and trephining of the skull, and even after the introduction of anaesthetics, results were poor until aseptic techniques became widely used.

e. Prognosis, or anticipation of the probable results of disease

As a science, prognosis, which must rest on numerical evidence, can hardly yet be said to exist. Clinical impressions have, of course, been recorded, but they have only recently begun to be submitted to critical scrutiny.

f. Palliation or alleviation of the effects of disease

If relief of both physical and mental suffering are included under palliation, this is certainly the oldest and was, at least until the nineteenth century, the most important medical service.

From the point of view of the public *a* and *b* are no more than means to the ends listed under *c–f*; and of these ends only the last (palliation) can be said to have been achieved before the nineteenth century. With the exception of vaccination against smallpox it seems unlikely that any specific measure of prevention or treatment was effective until the present century.

Although the analysis provided here is quite inadequate, a mere sketch of a subject which requires full and careful investigation, it is perhaps enough to show the lines such an inquiry might take and the type of conclusions to which it could lead. Apart from its intrinsic interest, an accurate assessment of medical work and achievement could have a powerful effect on contemporary thinking. It is instructive to learn that at all stages of history doctors have over-estimated the results of their intervention; to be reminded that diagnosis and understanding of disease are of no value to society until they lead to prevention or treatment; and to know that effective therapy was not available before the twentieth century and we must look elsewhere for an explanation of the large improvement in health which occurred earlier.

3. REASONS FOR IMPROVEMENT IN HUMAN HEALTH

Interpretation of improvement in health since the eighteenth century is among the most important subjects in history; yet so far it has had little attention from medical writers. Some have been interested in the decline of individual infectious diseases such as plague, smallpox, typhus, scarlet fever, and typhoid; but there have been few attempts to assess the contribution of medical and other influences to mortality as a whole, or the relation of mortality to the growth of population.

Investigation of the change in health leads inevitably to

consideration of population growth; but it is the modern rise of population as a whole which has to be explained, from some time in the eighteenth century when it began, until the present day. This subject deserves the fullest investigation, both in Britain and by extension to other countries where the increment in population and the time of changes such as industrialization were quite different. Until such inquiries have advanced to the point where their main conclusions are not in doubt, there will remain a serious deficiency in medical history and some difficult contemporary problems whose solution is prejudiced by lack of historical perspective.

4. THE EVOLUTION OF MEDICAL PRACTICE

The subjects so far discussed—influences on man's health, the tasks on which doctors have been engaged and the reasons for improvement in health—are all in a sense basic to a concept of human health and the part medicine and other influences play in preserving it. It is the lack of such insight which largely explains the misdirection of medical effort in the past, and the considerable confusion which still exists concerning the aims and methods of research and practice. This confusion is quite likely to increase, unless it is removed by the perspective the social history of medicine can uniquely provide. I want now to consider three other themes which illustrate the advantage of historical inquiry which takes as its starting point a contemporary problem. The first concerns medical practice.

There are few more important issues confronting medicine at the present time than the organization of medical practice. The fact that patterns of practice are very different in countries with a common language and similar social and political institutions suggests that medical practice has nowhere reached a satisfactory or stable form. For example, in some parts of Australia GPs have open access to hospitals and undertake services such as major surgery which would elsewhere be assigned to a specialist; in Britain, doctors are fairly sharply divided into GP and consultant classes, the one working outside and the other inside hospital; in the United States there are wide variations in the organization of practice, but in some areas GPs of the traditional type no longer exist and all services are provided by specialists.

There are some grounds for concern about all these patterns: in Australia about the quality of surgery and other specialist services provided by GPs; in Britain about the viability of general practice divorced from hospital; and in the United States about the loss of personal medical care outside hospital. Attempts are being made to meet some of the difficulties—for example all three countries are seeking to strengthen or reinstate family practice by GPs—but it is an open question whether they will succeed without more fundamental changes.

There are many subsidiary themes—the provision of home services, the use of the nurse or an assistant to the doctor in primary medical care, the need for personal care, the feasibility of family care and services in the patient's home are among them. But the central issue undoubtedly concerns the roles and relationships of the two major classes of medical worker—the GP and the consultant—and their respective functions in and out of hospitals. It is on this issue that I believe an examination of the evolution of medical practice can be illuminating.

A great deal of attention has been given by historians to such matters as the early history of the physician, surgeon, and apothecary, the founding of the Royal Colleges, and the events which led to the first Medical Act of 1858. But if the primary aim is to provide perspective on the contemporary problem, the focus of interest is quite different: it is on the circumstances which brought about the present pattern of practice. With this knowledge it may be possible to see whether the roles and relationship of GP and consultant were determined largely by fortuitous influences which have left their mark on the practice of medicine. It may be useful to summarize some tentative conclusions.

The history of physician, surgeon, and apothecary is well known, including the wide differences in their training, status, and types of practice. It was the building of hospitals during the eighteenth and nineteenth centuries that eroded these differences, and replaced them with a new distinction between those who had a hospital appointment and those who had not.

Although the trainings of physician, surgeon, and apothecary changed little during the eighteenth century, the traditional distinctions based on role and status began to break down. A sixteenth-century physician would have been horrified to be identified with a surgeon; but the new work in hospitals raised the status of the surgeon and the College of Surgeons received its Royal Charter in 1800. The important distinction was then between doctors who were appointed at the large voluntary hospitals, whether as physicians or surgeons, and those who were not.

At the same time the position of the apothecary was also changing. Although he had been visiting patients and prescribing for more than a century, it was not until 1703 that he was legally entitled to do so, provided he made no charge. During the eighteenth century he became established as the GP of the poor and middle classes. His training required six months' experience in hospital or dispensary and some apothecaries actually worked in hospitals. In the early nineteenth century the division between apothecaries and other practitioners was further diminished when some took a second qualification. It was no longer unknown for a doctor to practise legally as surgeon and apothecary, or even as physician and apothecary. This confusion of training, role, and status was part of the background of the 1858 Medical Act.

By providing a common basis for training and registration the Medical Acts of 1858 and 1886 finally removed the long-standing divisions between physician, surgeon, and apothecary. But by this time the new, and from a present-day viewpoint more significant, distinction between consultant and practitioner was well established. It was a distinction based, not on material differences in experience or competence, but on hospital appointments; the large voluntary hospitals in London and in the provinces were closed to the GP. There was indeed no true consultant, in the sense of one who sees only selected patients referred to him by other doctors, and in 1876 the *British Medical Journal* described the country consultant as 'the general practitioner who owes his position to the fact of his holding an appointment in connection with a country hospital'. The consultant was indeed little more than 'a practitioner among the rich', and according to the *Journal* the difference between the GP and the consultant really resolved itself into a difference of fees. It was not until the twentieth century that the state of medical knowledge really justified the emergence of a consultant class.

This preliminary examination of the evolution of the relationship between GP and consultant shows that this distinction began long before it was justified by the state of medical knowledge; it also suggests that the exclusion of GPs from hospital was not a logical development, but resulted from the fact that before the eighteenth century almost all practice was domiciliary, and as hospitals developed there was a strong competition for appointments in which, inevitably, not all were successful.

This knowledge of the evolution of medical practice, coupled with awareness of the wide variations which exist at the present time, helps us to approach the contemporary issues with open minds. It enables us to see that our pattern of practice is of relatively recent origin, that it was influenced largely by ephemeral circumstances and that the roles and relationship of GP and consultant should be reconsidered in the light of modern requirements and without assuming that what now exists is best because it is familiar.

5. THE HISTORY OF THE PUBLIC HEALTH SERVICE

The history of public health has been written very fully, but not in terms which throw much light on the problems which now confront the service. The central questions are its reorientation in countries where public responsibility has been accepted for all, or nearly all therapeutic as well as preventive services, and behind this the still larger issue of public competence and responsibility for administration of health services. In this context we turn to history for an understanding of the circumstances which determined the form, limitations, and local government control of public health rather than for a discussion of Acts of Parliament, the hypochondria of Florence Nightingale, or the removal of the handle of the Broad Street pump.

The introduction of environmental services by the 1848 Public Health Act raises two questions: one is why they were delayed so long, in view of measures such as quarantine and isolation which were taken centuries earlier; the other is why having been delayed they were established before, if only a short time before, the bacterial origin of infection was understood. A tentative answer to the first question is that the earlier measures were directed to epidemic rather than to endemic infections; and to the second, that public action was a sequel to ideas about the relationship between living conditions and health which had been developing since the early eighteenth century. Chadwick, in spite of his heresy concerning the nature of infectious disease, outlined very precisely the programme subsequently endorsed by bacteriologists: 'that the primary and most important measures, and at the same time the most practical, and within the recognized province of public administration, are drainage, the removal of all refuse from habitations, streets and roads, and the improvement of the supplies of water.' In this way, after about a million years' experience, men came to recognize the step which is second in importance or perhaps more accurately third, among measures which can be taken to improve human health.

The events which led local authorities to enter the field of personal health services soon after the beginning of this century are well known, not so much because they have attracted the interest of medical historians as because they are incorporated in the writings of the Fabians and particularly of the Webbs and Shaw. They publicized the extent of ill-health and the inadequacies of medical services, and enlivened the debate concerning the roles of private and public sectors in medical finance and administration. The issues then raised and the decisions concerning them were of outstanding importance and have left their mark on medical services to the present day.

Broadly there were two proposals: the one, that there should be a unified state medical service, based on public health principles and administered by local government; the other that the additional public services should be provided by doctors in private practice. The full implementation of either proposal might have prevented the division between preventive and treatment services, for the medical staffs of public health authorities were then extensively engaged in treatment as well as prevention of disease, and had both been sanctioned by Parliament, a unified service under local government would have resulted. Alternatively, had GPs been permitted to undertake the new work in schools and later in welfare clinics, the division might again have been avoided, and the later attitude of doctors to local authority administration and payment by salary might have been quite different. The compromise which made prevention a public responsibility and left cure in private hands had a profound impact on subsequent developments and, with the decision in 1911 not to assign National Health Insurance administration to local government, largely determined the framework which was retained in the NHS. It also led to the opposition of GPs and consultants to local authority administration of medical services.

The divided administration of local health services is, apparently, to be eliminated soon, at least in Britain; the large question concerning administration by elected or appointed bodies remains. In favour of local government it is said that the public which pays should manage the service; against, that experience of the public health service teaches that medical services are better in other hands. The answer to this question should turn on a penetrating analysis of the kinds of problems with which local health authorities have hitherto dealt and their degree of success in solving them. With this knowledge it would be possible to turn to the quite different problems which will present in the future, and to inquire whether in the light of past experience they should be assigned to local government or to appointed bodies. In the event the decision in Britain is likely to be taken on pragmatic grounds and it is questionable whether the efforts of social historians could have made a difference. But it certainly would be in the interests of many countries which have not passed the point of no return to see the history of public health in Britain written in relation to contemporary issues rather than in the traditional descriptive terms.

6. THE DEVELOPMENT OF HOSPITALS

It is hardly necessary to stress the importance of hospitals at the present time. They are the most costly component of medical services and the one whose expenditure is most difficult to control; they are the centres of research and training and have the influence derived from these activities; and since the arrangement of buildings and plant has a powerful influence on research and practice, they largely determine the direction of medical effort.

In Britain most hospitals date from the eighteenth and nineteenth centuries and now require substantial extension and reconstruction. It is essential that the new development should correct the mistakes of the past and, so far as possible, take account of future trends.

The most serious problems confronting hospitals derive from their fragmentation, particularly the separation of mental, chronic, and acute hospitals, but also the isolation of many acute facilities for patients such as women and children and for diseases such as those affecting the central nervous and cardiovascular systems. An examination of the historical development of hospitals explains these anomalies, attributing them to the joint influences of the casual way in which hospitals were founded, and the interpretation of their role which led acute hospitals to reject certain kinds of work.

Although the original purpose of the new hospitals founded by charity from the eighteenth century was to care for the sick poor, they soon began to admit only patients considered to be curable or, more accurately, likely to recover without treatment. They first excluded diseases such as infectious and venereal diseases, along with children and pregnant women, but by the mid nineteenth century admissions were largely restricted to short-term illness.

Some of the work rejected was taken up by other voluntary bodies; but there were three classes of patients which were beyond the means of voluntary bodies and largely outside the range of charitable appeal: the infectious, the mentally ill, and the destitute sick. Their exclusion led to a public hospital system and largely influenced its form.

Mental patients were the first for whom substantial public provision was made from 1808 when Parliament permitted (and later required) the building of county asylums for paupers. The founding of the second major division of the public hospital system was an unplanned consequence of revision of the Poor Law. The Amendment Act of 1834 was intended to end domiciliary aid by making it necessary for able-bodied paupers to enter an institution before they received public assistance. But in admitting the destitute, the Poor Law Authorities could not avoid admitting the sick, and by the end of the century most of the country's hospital beds were under the control of this unintended and ill-suited authority.

In recognition of the inadequacy of the Poor Law services, Parliament in 1867 authorized the construction of separate infirmaries, designed as hospitals and planned to follow the practices and, so far as possible, the standards of the voluntary hospitals. But the infirmaries also began to restrict admissions to acute cases and to accept patients above the pauper class. This meant that the formidable problem of caring for the indigent sick remained with the mixed workhouse, the institution least able to deal with it.

The other arm of the hospital service owed its origin to the failure of the voluntary hospitals to make provision for infectious disease. In 1867 Parliament authorized construction of fever hospitals and this led to the beginning of the municipal hospital system. At first it was concerned only with scarlet fever, enteric, typhus, and smallpox, but later the work was extended to include other fevers and, after the First World War, by addition of tuberculosis and maternity. Local sanitary authorities were also permitted to provide general hospitals but they had done so in only a few cases by 1929 when the functions of the

Poor Law authorities were transferred to the major local authorities.

This transfer reduced the number of hospital administrations to two, one public and the other private. It did not affect the widespread fragmentation of hospitals constructed during the eighteenth, nineteenth, and early twentieth centuries and still reflected in the haphazard services of every major town. Inadequate and badly located sites, hospitals too small to support essential services, and separation of related activities are the price that is still paid for the unplanned development. Their fragmentation is the origin of some of the most intractable problems confronting hospitals, including the division of work into favoured and depressed areas, staffing difficulties of mental chronic and some other hospitals, uneconomic management, and lack of flexibility in face of changing needs. Yet many people, including doctors, are still prepared to defend the traditional anomalies: small hospitals, fragmented facilities, and a division between acute and chronic services.

Historical research can make an invaluable contribution to correcting such misapprehensions, and indeed a rational approach to present and future hospital developments is hardly possible without it. But what is required for this purpose is not the traditional account of the history of individual hospitals, or the advances in medical knowledge with which they were associated, or the lives of the notable figures who have worked in them. All these subjects have their interest and it has been catered for generously in histories of medicine. The task which remains for the social historian is to interpret the evolution of hospitals against the background of the major problems which now confront them: provision of services of adequate standard for all classes of patients; rational accommodation to the uses and limitations of technology; reorientation of the services of teaching centres; restriction of costs; extension of research into neglected areas, particularly in the applied field. Without recognition of such problems the social history of medicine will be an esoteric study; and without historical perspective medical science and service will continue to drift.

Discussion

Many historians of medicine have been physicians who have approached their subject against a background of clinical experience. This was not necessarily undesirable; indeed it served a purpose in so far as it provided a basis for the understanding of clinical problems. However, the approach of some social historians has been different; they tend to start from a sociocentric rather than from an iatrocentric viewpoint. This viewpoint may be expressed as follows. A society has health problems which are related to social organization and living conditions. Attempts are made to solve these problems, and lead to the development of medical traditions which are a function of social activity and social organization. This of course suffers from over-simplification since there can be no denying the fact that the origins of social medicine are clinical.

Trevelyan described social history as history with the politics left out. Many social historians would today reject this definition; since social history deals with man in his social and institutional environment, it cannot fail to be concerned with his political history as well as with his social and economic history.

To deal with these matters from a historical viewpoint requires knowledge of the people, their health problems, and their medical and social institutions. Here one must be careful not to denigrate earlier achievements, and it is salutary to recall E. M. Forster's comment in his essay on *The Consolations of History*: 'It is pleasant to be transferred from an office where one is afraid of a sergeant major into an office where one can intimidate generals. This is perhaps why history is so attractive to the more timid among us. We can recover self-confidence by snubbing the dead.'

It is also important to judge earlier developments in their own context rather than on present-day terms. The Code of Hammurabi reflects the social structure of Babylonia as accurately as that of the American Medical Association reflects a contemporary ethical viewpoint. Moreover since history is dynamic, experience should be seen at two points in time, the one when it occurred and the other at some later date when the changes can be assessed.

Many people have been convinced that it is possible to learn from history, and this conclusion is acceptable so long as certain cautions are exercised. One is to recognize that while men make their own history, the way in which they do so is influenced by the circumstances in which they find themselves, and these are determined largely by the past. For example, the different developments of medical practice in Australia, Britain, and the USA were not fortuitous but are attributable to differences in the environments in which they arose. The strong tendency towards private and individual medical practice in the USA is related to the separate control of licensing and practice by each of fifty states, while in Britain the more uniform medical profession was associated with the more homogeneous setting in which it developed. Specialization has taken quite different forms in Britain, the USA, and elsewhere, forms largely determined by social, economic, and other influences. The history of public health in the nineteenth century might also be used to illustrate the extent to which medical developments were affected by public as well as professional attitudes and circumstances. Used in this way, history does more than provide background and perspective; it enables us to understand past trends which in a sense have determined the present. History does not teach what should be done, but it makes men more prudent and helps them to recognize the choices that are open to them.

The opening paper outlined an operational approach to the study of history, based on prior identification of a contemporary problem on which historical insight is sought. Used judiciously this method is of value, particularly where it leads to hypotheses which can be confirmed or rejected on the basis of historical evidence. It is possible to use a comparative method. For example, the community approach in the USA is leading to the creation of neighbourhood health or medical centres. Centres of this type were established fifty years ago, and it is of value to know the history of the earlier development. In this way history, used pragmatically, can be of considerable assistance in contemporary planning.

At the same time it should be recognized that history is of interest in its own right and does not require to be justified wholly by its utility. Moreover, it is by no means the only evidence which is relevant to present-day problems and in some cases it may be quite irrelevant. Nevertheless the theme of the Symposium is 'Medical History and Medical Care' and it is those areas in which historical insight can assist contemporary planning that are of particular interest.

One of these areas is medical education and the following memoir on the changes which have taken place since the beginning of the twentieth century in the USA opened a discussion on the factors influencing certain changes in the characteristics of the profession.

Changes in the supply and characteristics of American doctors in the twentieth century[1]

JOHN Z. BOWERS

I shall focus my remarks on some of the changes in the supply and characteristics of American doctors that have profoundly affected medical care during the present century. In preparing this comment, I have benefited from reading an excellent recent analysis of developments in medical education and medical care in the USA in this century by Dr Julius Richmond (9).

By 1900 a large number of doctors were being trained in the USA and a favourable physician/population ratio existed. The majority were being trained (one could hardly say educated) in mediocre to bad, privately owned medical schools.

The first true graduate school, that at Johns Hopkins, was not opened until 1876—prior to that time students in most fields had to go abroad for their graduate studies. Medical graduates went to Vienna, Leipzig, Berlin, and other great European medical centres for their further training.

This situation was well described in 1910 by a scholarly observer: 'For twenty-five years there has been an enormous over-production of uneducated and ill trained medical practitioners . . . due in the main to the existence of a very large number of commercial schools, sustained in many cases by advertising methods through which a mass of unprepared youth is drawn out of industrial occupations to the study of medicine' (8).

1. A memoir by Dr Bowers based on remarks made at the opening session.

First let us consider some of the sociological influences that led to the drastic reform of medical education in the USA that followed the 'Flexner Report'.

The first decade of the twentieth century was characterized by a striking development in national resources, character, and pride. This enrichment was largely due to the leadership of President Theodore Roosevelt, who held office from 1901 to 1909. It may be said that George Washington founded the nation, that Lincoln preserved it, and that Theodore Roosevelt revitalized it. In such a climate of change, new life was instilled into a wide variety of existing institutions, including education, and new institutions were established. 'Trust busting' was the theme of the day; there could hardly have been a trust more deserving of busting than medicine. Indeed, some have speculated that the trust-busting atmosphere may have influenced Andrew Carnegie and John D. Rockefeller to establish the philanthropies that largely made possible the reform of medical education in the USA. This is not to deny that within the medical profession cries of concern were issuing from the Council of Medical Education of the American Medical Association. However, these voices alone were not capable of instigating the radical reform that was essential.

Fortunately, a few men of great wealth were following the examples set by Sir Thomas Bodley in his benefaction to Oxford in 1602 and by Sir Thomas Guy in 1724 in founding a hospital in London.[1] They were Andrew Carnegie, a Scot, who, among his many benefactions, established the Carnegie Foundation for the Advancement of Teaching in 1905, and John D. Rockefeller who, two years earlier, in 1903, had founded the General Education Board. The Carnegie Foundation, as one aspect of its programme, became interested in the improvement of professional education in the USA. Religiosity was a dominant social force in the USA in those years, leading Henry Allen Moe to comment: 'Religion is the mother of philanthropy' (7). Both Mr Carnegie and Mr Rockefeller were deeply religious men; Mr Rockefeller's principal advisor was a Baptist minister, the Revd Frederick T. Gates.

There are differences of opinion as to the exact role of the American Medical Association in the decision of the Carnegie Foundation to undertake the study of medical education in the USA, but we need not enter that discussion here (see 1, 2, 3, 4; for the AMA viewpoint see 5, 6).

The story of the Flexner Report has been told many times and need not be repeated here. It is interesting to note, however, that a

1. Guy's wealth was 'derived from South Sea Stock speculations which had brought scandal and bankruptcy to others' (10).

singular confluence of philanthropic interests gave Abraham Flexner the opportunity by which he made such an important contribution. Having completed his study, he was asked by Frederick Gates what should be done to implement it. Flexner responded by joining the staff of the General Education Board and launching a programme that ultimately gave $78 million to twenty-four medical schools. How many other 'studies' or 'reports', or even 'Royal Commissions', have had such an opportunity and have achieved so much?

As a result of the Flexner Report, there was a sharp fall in the number of new doctors: from 5,700 graduates in 1900 to 2,300 graduates in 1919. One-third of the nation's medical schools were closed. Dr Julius Richmond has speculated that if more of the non-university affiliated schools had continued to operate, the production of practitioners would have been greater and the distribution of medical care might have been more satisfactory (9).

Doctors in the USA are more attached to the private practice of medicine than are physicians in any other country save for those in Latin America and the Philippines, and the continuing and unfortunate antagonism of the American Medical Association toward government-sponsored medicine is well known. This situation has been and is to a large extent based on financial factors. The question frequently asked in the USA is: 'Why are doctors so avaricious?' One reason is that many leading practitioners entered the profession during the great depression. Those lean years were soon followed by another period of low income during the Second World War, making a total span of fifteen years of low income.

Another reason stems from the fact that, although residency programmes extended increasingly the time of training following the internship, there was no adequate financial support during these spans and many young physicians entering practice were deeply in debt. Many men who had married and whose wives had worked to support them were eager to enjoy the 'good life' with their families.

When medical schools made efforts to extend their medical care activities outside the walls of their teaching hospitals, they encountered strong opposition from practitioners who feared that they would suffer financial loss from the competition. Indeed, many teaching hospitals, especially those attached to state-supported schools, were permitted to accept only those patients referred by a practitioner.

The extraordinary growth of medical research in the USA was fostered by 'medical research lobbies', composed of citizens, politicians, and scientists. The first major thrust was directed at poliomyelitis by a private agency that was founded as a tribute to a political leader, President Franklin D. Roosevelt, himself a victim of polio and a constant public reminder of the potential ravages of this disease. Emphasis in the medical schools was on 'bench' research and on patient-oriented studies of hospitalized patients conducted in clinical research centres.

The departments of preventive medicine that might have become centres for the study of medical care were in a 'search for identity', were seriously under-financed, and were frequently 'mini' departments of microbiology or internal medicine. Schools of public health were mainly concerned with epidemiology and public health administration. One should not overly condemn these faculties, however, because the available money went into biomedical research, and the schools naturally went where they could find financial support.

The years since 1960 have seen a slowly but steadily increasing concern for the development of medical care programmes in schools of medicine and public health. Governmental and citizen forces have challenged these schools to expedite the application of new knowledge to the patient.

Finally, one should note the increasing effect of 'student force' on medical care programmes in the USA. Today's medical students have a deep concern for the poor, for social justice, and for racial equality. The number of medical students aspiring to careers in curative and preventive health services has risen sharply. Weller reports: 'Whereas four years ago 4 per cent of students entering Harvard Medical School indicated that public health was their career objective, this year 39 per cent of entering students state that public health is their first or second choice for a career' (11). They insist that the faculties develop outlets by which these concerns may be implemented. Their voices have become important and constructive, albeit at times troublesome, forces in turning the eyes of the faculty from the hospital bed to medical care services in community. It is no exaggeration to state that an area heretofore largely ignored has become the central focus of current attention.

REFERENCES

1. Flexner, Abraham (1940). *I Remember* (New York).

2. —— (1943). *Henry S. Pritchett: A Biography* (New York: Columbia).

3. —— (1952). *Funds and Foundations: Their Policies, Past and Present* (with the collaboration of Esther S. Bailey) (Harper).

4. Gregg, Alan (1947). 'On Abraham Flexner's eightieth birthday', *J. hist. Med.* 2, 487–8.

5. Johnson, Victor (1947). 'The Council on Medical Education and Hospitals', in Fishbein, Morris, *A History of the American Medical Association, 1876–1947* (Philadelphia: W. B. Saunders Co.), pp. 887–922.

6. —— (1964). 'Self-discipline in medical education', *The Pharos* (July), 73–82.

7. MOE, H. A. (1961). *Proceedings of the American Philosophical Society*, 105 (April), no. 2, p. 141.

8. PRITCHETT, HENRY S. (1910). Introduction in Flexner, Abraham, *Medical Education in the United States and Canada: A Report to the Carnegie Foundation for the Advancement of Teaching*, Bulletin no. 4, p. x (New York City) (also quoted by Richmond).

9. RICHMOND, JULIUS B. (1969). *Currents in American Medicine: A Developmental View of Medical Care and Education* (Cambridge: Harvard University Press).

10. WEAVER, WARREN (1967). *U.S. Philanthropic Foundations: Their History, Structure, Management, and Record* (New York, Evanston, and London: Harper and Row).

11. WELLER, T. H. (1970). 'Medical research as "measured against the needs of all"', Editorial, *New Eng. J. of Med.* 283, no. 10, 537–9.

Discussion

Currently one of the most important issues in medical care throughout the world is the shortage of doctors. This is a relatively recent phenomenon and reflects two things: first, the great advances in medicine which require more manpower; and second, the greater demand for more services. The effect has been a massive expansion in medical education.

In Britain there is a sharp division of opinion in education between the élitists, who feel that more means worse, and the others who feel strongly that more, in fact, means better. There is, however, a belief strongly held that there is now better training, better motivation, and on the whole better medical education than ever before.

Not only have medical schools expanded, however, but a significant change that has occurred in Britain in the last quarter of a century especially is a broadening of the social base from which the medical profession is recruited. This can be traced to the universal application of student grants.

The effect of student grants in Britain has been completely to alter the social background of doctors. In the civic universities, although there is a relatively small number of the sons and daughters of manual workers, there is a very massive recruitment from the lower and middle, middle class. Without the grant system much potential talent would be lost simply because a lot of people could not afford to go to medical school.

Traditionally in the past those with no scientific background but with a classical or historical background were freely admitted to the medical school, but the emphasis on scientific medicine and the extreme competition for places in medical schools have meant there is now a premium on preparation in the more scientific subjects.

To the English observer the fees in American medical schools appear astronomical, which with the cost of maintenance would seem to restrict both the number and the social orientation of the doctors recruited. Comparing the experience of both systems it is difficult not to speculate on how long the medical profession can be recruited in realistic numbers in the USA without a measure of public support for recruits from a much wider social range.

It was pointed out, however, that in the USA there is considerable variation in costs; and those schools with state support tend to have lower tuition costs and fees than the private institutions. Increasingly as the recruitment of students is widened to include those from minority groups or from underprivileged backgrounds, states have authorized the waiving of tuition fees—another form, of course, of public support.

With regard to the social structure from which medical students are drawn, hitherto this has been predominantly middle and upper class; but medical schools are increasingly seeking to recruit medical students from the minority groups, principally Negroes, a policy which is bringing about a completely new perspective. Yet it must be conceded it is going to be difficult to develop such a policy effectively without considerable public support. While encouraging the general movement, the present administration seems to be favouring a movement towards loans, away from scholarships. Many schools in the USA have rather extensive private funds available for scholarships and for loans.

There is, of course, more to it than just the financial side. There is also the question of preparation through general education. Many of the students who might come from the lower social classes or groups do not come, simply because they have not had the necessary basic education. This is a problem which has been recognized but upon which not enough has been really done so far. The student has to graduate from the secondary school and the college systems to be able to get into the medical school, and many of them, often for social reasons, cannot achieve these intermediate goals. Yet many schools have accepted minority students—students with what would be ordinarily considered to be an inadequate background, and special tutorial help is given.

An instance was given of how Stanford University has had just such a policy for some years, of taking suitable students who otherwise would not have qualified for entry. In summarizing the records of these people, their over-all averages have on the whole been better than the Stanford undergraduate body as a whole. One must conclude from this that some of the original fears seem to be not fully grounded. It is true that the problems in medicine are a little different. Yet in the medical school from the experience hitherto it appears that many of these students, despite the disability of poor background, are getting on very well and there is likely to be a great increase in numbers of such students in the future, particularly if financial aid can be made available.

Indeed the number of minority Negro students entering American medical schools was 200 two years ago, 450 one year ago, and it was close to 700 in 1970. This indicates how the situation is changing fast. The problem is to make medical education broadly available to those in the general spectrum of society who wish to do it and who are in fact qualified for it.

Of course, this is in the perspective of a general policy for minority groups and is unlikely to apply to a mass of lower middle-class boys and girls who would probably be attracted to medicine if the financial situation were generally different. All countries will probably be forced to take note of this in the end and have some policy to obviate the difficulties because obviously if not they will be failing to draw talent from an important section of the population.

2

A HISTORICAL APPRAISAL OF THE MEDICAL TASK

THOMAS McKEOWN

A historical appraisal of the medical task

Historians recognize that scientific advance is influenced largely by the way in which problems are formulated, and that discoveries may be delayed long after the requisite technical basis becomes available, by failure in conceptualization. Crombie cites as an example the first major development in modern physiology, Kepler's discovery in 1604 of the dioptric mechanism by which the eye produces the retinal image (1). The technical knowledge needed for this advance was available in second-century Alexandria, but the Greek's 'formulation of the problem did not allow them to see in the eye itself a subject for optical analysis'.

The approach to biology and medicine established during the seventeenth century was an engineering one based on a physical model. Nature was conceived in mechanistic terms, which led in biology to the idea that a living organism could be regarded as a machine which might be taken apart and reassembled if its structure and function were fully understood. In medicine the same concept led further to the belief that an understanding of disease processes and of the body's response to them would make it possible to intervene therapeutically, mainly by physical (surgical), chemical, or electrical methods. Psychiatry is thought to be backward because it has only recently begun to use these methods, but this is attributed to the difficulties of the subject or the deficiencies of its practitioners rather than to any inherent difference which would make it necessary to modify the approach. In population biology the mechanistic interpretation has been enlarged by statistical concepts, but in medicine these have not yet significantly altered the attack, statistics being used to determine the most appropriate therapeutic intervention rather than to provide any new conceptualization derived from a different model.

The consequences of the engineering approach are even more conspicuous in medicine today than they were in the seventeenth century largely because the resources of the physical and chemical sciences are so much greater. Medical education begins with the study of the structure and function of the body, continues with examination of disease processes, and ends with clinical instruction on selected sick people; medical service is dominated by the image of the acute hospital where the technological resources are concentrated; and medical science reflects the mechanistic concept, for example in the attention given to the chemical basis of inheritance and the immunological response to transplanted organs. These researches are strictly in accord with the physical model, the first being thought to lead ultimately to control of gene structure and the second to replacement of diseased organs by normal ones.

In the present context the question is not whether the engineering approach is predominant in medicine, which would hardly be disputed, but whether it is seriously deficient as a conceptualization of the problems of human health. An answer will be sought in two ways: by assessing the reasons for the transformation of health which has occurred since the eighteenth century; and by evaluating the major influences on the health of living things and the special problems which arise in their application to man.

REASONS FOR IMPROVEMENT IN HEALTH

Historical interpretation of changes in health must rely largely on knowledge of the behaviour of the death-rate and the contribution made to it by different causes of death. In Britain this information is available from 1838; but the fact that the population increased rapidly during the previous century suggests that mortality may have declined well before the rate was first recorded. Hence assessment of the reasons for improvement in health leads inescapably to consideration of the modern rise of population.

That there has been so far no convincing interpretation is not wholly attributable to the difficulties of the subject. Medical historians have largely ignored it, though many of the issues which it raises are medical; and economic historians, being primarily interested in the relation between population growth and the Industrial Revolution, have focused their attention on the earlier and, in view of the paucity of data, more difficult phase. There have been few attempts to look at the growth of population as a whole, and to provide an explanation which considers both birth-rate and death-rate, and takes account not only of medical measures, but also of the vast agricultural and industrial changes in the eighteenth and nineteenth centuries.

For a comprehensive interpretation of the rise of population there is no more important decision than the choice of methods by which it is to be investigated. The essential requirement for this is information concerning birth-rate, death-rate, and cause of death; this is not available nationally before 1838 and it is questionable whether data from other sources such as parish registers can provide a substitute in the pre-registration years. If this conclusion is correct, it is better to examine post-registration evidence before turning to the uncertainties in the eighteenth century, when the modern rise of population began.

Population growth after registration

National statistics show that from 1838 the growth of population was due to an existing excess of births over deaths, supported later by a decline of mortality. Since the time when birth-rate and death-rate were reliably recorded there is no evidence of a rising birth-rate in England and Wales, or in other European countries, including Scandinavia where the records begin in the mid eighteenth century. Indeed in respect of the modern rise of population as a whole it is more accurate to say that it occurred in spite of a decrease of the birth-rate rather than because of an increase.

There is also no doubt that from the time when cause of death was first registered, the decline of mortality was due to a reduction of deaths from communicable disease. This was certainly true in the nineteenth and early twentieth centuries and national statistics show that even in recent years the decrease in the death-rate has resulted mainly from control of the infections.

There is probably little disagreement about the interpretation to this point and it is hard to see that there should be difficulty over the further conclusion that until the second quarter of the twentieth century the decline of mortality from infections owed little to specific measures of preventing or treating disease in the individual. Mortality began to fall before identification of the causal organisms and, with the exception of smallpox whose contribution to the total reduction was small, long before the introduction of effective immunization or treatment.

The only specific reasons for a substantial decline of mortality that can be identified during the nineteenth century were the hygienic measures introduced progressively from about 1870 (2). Improvements in water supplies and sewage disposal began at that time, and the fact that they coincided with a decline of mortality from intestinal infections provides good evidence of their effectiveness.

However there had been a large reduction of deaths from tuberculosis between 1840 and 1870 and some other explanation must be sought for it. After reviewing the evidence McKeown and Record attributed the decline of mortality to a rising standard of living, in particular to improvements in nutrition (2). This conclusion is in accord with that reached by Hart and Wright after detailed consideration of tuberculosis (3).

In summary, the increase of population after 1838 was due to an excess of births over deaths established by the time of registration, supported later by a further decline of mortality. The main reasons for the decline, in order of time and magnitude, were (*a*) an improvement in standard of living, particularly of nutrition, (*b*) hygienic measures form about 1870, and

(c) prevention and treatment of disease in the individual from the second quarter of the present century.

The rise of population before registration will be considered in the light of this interpretation for the later period.

Population growth before registration

In Britain it is not possible to state precisely when the modern rise in population began; but it was well established before registration of births and deaths, and even at the time of the first census (1801) the increase in numbers was much greater than in previous centuries. Hence there is no doubt that the expansion started during the eighteenth century.

The reasons for the early phase of population growth can be examined under three headings: medical measures of preventing or treating disease in the individual, leading to a decline of mortality; a spontaneous reduction of mortality from infectious disease; and improvement in the standard of living, whether leading to an increase of the birth-rate or decrease of the death-rate. This approach, suggested by prior consideration of the post-registration period, makes the relative importance of birth-rate and death-rate, the issue which has had so much attention from economic historians, secondary to the larger question: what disturbed either rate?

With the single exception of vaccination against smallpox there is no specific medical measure which can be seen to have influenced the trend of mortality from an infectious disease before the twentieth century. Smallpox made only a small contribution to the reduction of the national death-rate after registration, and since vaccination came into use after 1800 it would seem to follow that prevention or treatment of disease had no effect on mortality before that time (2). The suggestion that the crude procedure of inoculation with infected material was responsible for a reduction of the national death-rate in the eighteenth century has convinced few if any medical writers, least of all virologists who know smallpox (4, 5). In addition to their specific objections, based on extensive personal experience, there is the further point that the trend of national mortality over a considerable period is most unlikely to be explained by the behaviour of a single disease. Even the most effective of the vaccines now available, if used in the eighteenth century could not be expected to have had the influence recently ascribed to the crude and dangerous practice of inoculation.

There is no reason to question that one or more infections may have declined spontaneously in the eighteenth century, like scarlet fever in later periods, and the disappearance of plague has been suggested as a possible, though entirely unsupported, explanation for population changes (6). However, it cannot account for the unprecedented increase of numbers between 1700 and 1840, an increase which began a hundred years before sanitary reform and a hundred and fifty years before significant medical intervention.

Exclusion of medical measures and of a large spontaneous reduction of mortality leaves a third possible explanation for the increase of population before registration, namely an improvement in standard of living. In his Presidential Address to the British Association, Hutchinson suggested that the standard of living rose because of advances in British agriculture (7). He quoted Ernle: 'In 1811 (the population of England and Wales) had grown to 10,150,615. On these figures the population had doubled itself in 125 years and even if no allowance is made for an improved standard of living, it is probable that England during the same period had doubled her production of food' (8). Hutchinson states that by the end of the Napoleonic Wars production had outstripped consumption, and it was not until the 1870s that imported food from North America began to make a significant contribution.

The suggestion that the most important influence on population growth during the eighteenth and early nineteenth centuries was an increase in home-grown food supplies may be thought to reopen the question whether the initial impetus to population growth was a rise of the birth-rate or a fall of the death-rate. It is not a question which need be considered in detail here; what is hardly in doubt is that the difference between the birth- and death-rate established before the time of registration

(1838) must have been due largely to a substantial decline of mortality from infectious disease.

The importance attached to food supplies raises a further question: Why should an improvement in man's nutrition be a disaster for infectious organisms? or, to put the point more specifically, if less colourfully: Why should better nutrition tip the balance in favour of host over parasite? The conclusions which follow are based on Andrewes's discussion of the evolution of viruses, extrapolated to micro-organisms in general (9).

Most micro-organisms do not harm their hosts and in some cases the association is mutually beneficial. The circumstances under which disease occurs include the following.

(*a*) When induced disease assists the spread of the organism. Andrewes cites the 'coughs and sneezes' which distribute the cold virus and the encephalitis from rabies which makes dogs bite other animals. Other examples are diarrhoea associated with cholera and coughing from respiratory tuberculosis which assist the spread of bacteria.

(*b*) When the host–parasite equilibrium is disturbed in favour of the parasite, for example in pure strains of herds or crops which facilitate spread and increase in virulence of infective organisms.

(*c*) The spread of a micro-organism to a new host, which may lead to sickness and death (of host or parasite) before equilibrium is established.

These mechanisms suggest an answer to the question posed at the beginning of this brief discussion of the relation between nutrition and infectious disease. Most micro-organisms are harmless to their hosts and probably benefited from the larger and healthier population which resulted from increased food supplies; it is therefore incorrect to conclude that improved nutrition was a disaster for them. But in the case of certain organisms which cause disease, the improvement tipped the balance in favour of the host over the parasite. It is more likely to have done so in some of the chronic diseases such as tuberculosis referred to under (*a*) above, where nutritional state is known to be important, than in the case of acute epidemic infections such as smallpox or measles referred to under (*c*), whose distribution is largely independent of social and economic conditions.

This interpretation of the modern rise of population puts the emphasis on a rising standard of living, particularly improved food supplies from 1770 or earlier, removal of adverse influences in the physical environment by hygienic measures from about 1870, and specific preventive and therapeutic measures from the second quarter of the twentieth century. However in time, and on an evolutionary scale a fairly short time, those advances would again have been overtaken by increasing numbers if population growth had not been brought under control by the decline of the birth-rate. If the birth-rate in England and Wales had remained at the level of 1870, the population today would be 140 million instead of 46 million, with effects on standards of living and health that can be imagined .

Thus experience of England and Wales is consistent with Malthus's thesis. Although the improvement in health was initiated by increased food supplies, without limitation of numbers the advance would soon have been eliminated. Viewed historically, the balance between food and population size on which health depends owes less to increase of food than to control of numbers.

It is concluded that in order of importance the major contributions to improvement in health in England and Wales were from limitation of family size (a behavioural change), increase in food supplies and a healthier physical environment (environmental influences), and specific preventive and therapeutic measures.

INFLUENCES ON HEALTH

The preceding discussion led to the conclusion that in England and Wales medical measures derived from the engineering approach to man's health have been much less important than a change in reproductive behaviour, provision of food, and removal of adverse influences from the environment. But the experience of the past two centuries was unique in some respects which have a bearing on this problem: for example in the occurrence of the Agricultural and Industrial Revolutions; in the beginning of extensive control of human reproduction; in the discovery of the nature of infectious disease; and in the introduction of effective methods of preventing and treating disease in the individual patient. It might perhaps be argued that as the period was unique, so to were the reasons for improved health within it, and that on a longer appraisal in more varied conditions the main influences might prove to be quite different. Indeed there is already evidence that at least the timing has changed in developing countries, where the application of specific environmental measures has preceded an improvement in the standard of living.

In order to come to a conclusion about the general acceptability of the interpretation outlined above it is possible to examine the major influences on the health of living things and the circumstances which restrict their application to man. The discussion will be concerned mainly with animals, though many of the conclusions would be equally true of plants.

The key to the riddle presented by the health of living things lies in the relation of reproduction to mortality. Both have evolved through natural selection; but they have not evolved in balance, in the sense that numbers born are restricted in relation to the numbers that can survive. Wynne-Edwards has presented a contrary view, that animals limit their numbers largely by social behaviour and biological restraints on reproduction (10). However, this interpretation has been challenged strongly by Lack and since it has no relevance to human populations it will not be considered further (11).

An alternative, and I believe more convincing interpretation, suggests that the size of natural populations is controlled by density-dependent mortality. In wild birds and some other animals (Lack mentions carnivorous mammals, certain rodents, large fish where not fished, and a few insects) the level of mortality is determined mainly by the availability of food. However, there are other animals, possibly many more in which, though numbers are limited ultimately by food supplies, these limits are not usually reached because population size is restricted by predators, including insect parasites, and disease.

On this interpretation, the essential requirements for reduction of mortality and improvement in health of animal populations are (*a*) equating of food supplies and population size, by increasing the amount of food and limiting numbers by control of reproduction and (*b*) removal of other causes of mortality, particular predators, including in some cases human predators, and parasites.

This theoretically derived programme is in accord with what has actually happened in domestication of both animals and plants. Their numbers and distribution are controlled; more and better food is provided, manure and fertilizers for plants, foodstuffs in a variety of forms for animals; and domesticated plants and animals are protected as far as possible from environmental hazards, including parasites, predators, and severe weather.

Another method of outstanding importance in domestication has been selective breeding. This has been used to accentuate characters desired by man, sometimes with side effects on health from production of pure strains which may increase the spread and virulence of micro-organisms. But cross-breeding has also been used to produce hardier stocks by heterosis.

These measures which have been predominant in plant and animal husbandry are essentially population methods and owe little to the engineering approach. It is fairly obvious why little use has been made of physical or chemical manipulation of individual plants or animals. In the first place, except in the case of pets and unique specimens such as race-horses and prize cattle, man has little interest in individual examples of species other than his own. Secondly, it is much more economical to deal with large numbers in preference to identifying and manipulating single specimens. And finally, a conclusion which is particularly relevant to the problems of human health, population methods are far more effective than individual methods. Indeed when they are fully applied there is little need for an engineering approach, for under adequately controlled conditions the large majority of those born alive remain healthy.

In relation to health how far is it possible to extrapolate from other animals to man? Until the eighteenth century the human situation was essentially the same as that of other natural populations. Numbers born were greatly in excess of numbers that could survive, and population size was limited by density-dependent mortality. (Until the eighteenth century there is no evidence of restriction of population size, either by deliberate control of reproduction or by the instinctive restraints of the kind suggested by Wynne-Edwards in other animals [10].) The high level of mortality was due mainly to starvation, disease, and self-destruction by war or homicide.

With one important reservation, the methods of improving human health are identical to those which are applicable to other animals. Like other living things, man has been exposed to rigorous natural selection, and the majority of those born alive are healthy in the sense that they are adapted to the environment in which they live. His primary need is for sufficient food, which requires both an increase in food supplies and limitation of numbers. But he also needs protection from certain hazards in the physical environment; over any considerable period disease due to micro-organisms was probably the most important, though at times homicide, the human analogue of predation, was also very significant.

The notable difference between human and other animal experience in relation to health, results from the ethical restraints which prohibit control of reproduction. But human beings are uniquely educable, and can learn voluntarily to limit family size. In this way a behavioural change may achieve the same result as the restrictions imposed by man on other animals.

In summary, to achieve good health, man, like other animals requires sufficient food, limitation of numbers, and protection from hazards in the physical environment. He differs only in this, that control of reproduction and avoidance of external risks such as injury or death by war, have to be learned rather than imposed. Given these advantages, his need for physical or chemical intervention with the functions of the body is not great.

This conclusion is in accord with the interpretation suggested for the improvement in health since the eighteenth century. This is not to say that wherever human health improves, the timing will invariably be the same as that in England and Wales. Indeed two exceptions are already well documented: in France the reduction of the birth-rate was much earlier than in the British Isles, and preceded control of the physical environment by sanitary measures; and in developing countries today, economical and effective sanitary measures such as spraying against insects are preceding both control of numbers and a general improvement in the standard of living and nutrition. These changes in timing do not affect the conclusions concerning the major influences, all of which are needed to achieve the levels of health already attained in some parts of the world.

RESIDUAL HEALTH PROBLEMS

The discussion to this point was concerned with the basic requirements for health in natural populations, exposed to the hazards which probably existed throughout man's evolution. But health problems have been transformed in technologically advanced countries, and it is conceivable that the major influences are now quite different from those of the past. In particular, the possibility should be considered that specific measures of preventing and treating disease derived from the engineering approach are relatively more important in populations with long expectation of life and largely protected from the threat of infectious disease.

First, it should be noted that the contribution of the traditional measures is far from being exhausted. It is questionable whether the growth of population has been anywhere restricted to a rate commensurate with modern health, welfare, and recreational requirements. Incredibly, in some of the most advanced countries, there are substantial sections of the population which are inadequately (as distinct from unwisely) fed. In all countries there remain significant environmental hazards, such as accidents, atmospheric pollution, and defective housing. And finally the threat of war is nowhere removed, while the risks to health if it occurs are immeasurably increased.

Nevertheless the improvements of the past two centuries have greatly altered the character of the predominant health problems. Given effective application of the traditional methods, a large majority of those who are not congenitally handicapped can expect to remain healthy until late life if they are not affected by mental illness. This is merely another and possibly more obscure way of saying that in technologically advanced countries the residual health problems are mainly congenital, psychiatric, and geriatric. Since the problems presented by these three types of illness are quite different, they must be considered separately in order to assess whether the major influences on health have also changed.

Congenital disability

While there has been some improvement, indicated by the decline of stillbirth and neonatal mortality rates, congenital causes of sickness, disability, and death have been relatively unresponsive to the influences which have been so effective postnatally. There has been no significant reduction of the incidence of such major handicaps as mental defect and congenital malformations, and most deaths between conception and the end of childhood are now determined prenatally.

These findings are not difficult to explain. Fertilization, implantation, and early embryonic development are hazardous processes, in which occasional mistakes are inevitable and often serious. The intra-uterine location largely protects the foetus from external hazards, but also means that it is unlikely to benefit greatly from their removal. For the same reason the abnormal foetus is relatively inaccessible to physical or chemical intervention.

Within that part of the future which it is realistic to discuss, there is little prospect of reducing substantially the incidence of congenital diseases and disabilities either by some miracle of genetic engineering or by contraception requiring identification of parents whose offspring will be affected. In most cases correction of abnormalities by intra-uterine intervention is also unlikely. The only effective approach to the problem presented by most serious congenital handicaps is their recognition during pregnancy and elimination by abortion.

There is considerable scope for improvement of obstetric care before and during delivery. But this is for the purpose of protecting the mother and normal foetus during birth rather than of correcting the disability of the abnormal one.

This short appraisal suggests that the measures likely to be effective with congenital diseases and disabilities are quite different from those which have been successful in post-natal life. They depend largely on direct intervention, the recognition and removal of the abnormal embryo or foetus, and obstetric care before and during labour to ensure the safe delivery of a normal child. This is not to say that in relation to pregnancy and birth adequate food and a safe environment are no longer important. But when these essentials can be taken for granted, as they largely can in favoured sections of the populations of technologically advanced countries, the solution of the congenital problems which remain will depend on measures which can be said to derive from the engineering approach.

However, it should also be recognized that the time is not yet in sight when this approach will make it possible to prevent the birth of most seriously handicapped children. In the immediate future, the care, rather than the abortion of the mentally defective and the malformed, to mention only the most common of the serious handicaps, will remain the predominant feature of the task presented by the congenitally disabled.

Mental illness

Opinion is so widely divided about the nature of mental illness that it is unrealistic to expect agreement about the measures on which its control will depend. The gap is immeasurable between the psycho-analysts and those who believe it is practicable to seek a physical or chemical solution of psychiatric problems. Nevertheless some points which have a bearing on this issue are probably not in dispute.

One is that the major forms of mental illness have not responded to the measures which have been so effective in reducing mortality. The virtual disappearance of tertiary syphilis, once a common cause of admission to psychiatric hospitals, is the best-documented exception, and there is little doubt that illnesses associated with nutritional and toxic causes have also declined. But with such exceptions the common forms of neurotic, psychotic, and psychosomatic illness appear to be at least as prevalent as formerly.

A second point of possible agreement is that the volume and types of psychiatric and psychosomatic illness may differ considerably in different populations and in the same population at different times. Remarkable examples are the variation in incidence of peptic ulcer in countries of western Europe, and the change in the male to female ratio of deaths due to perforation from peptic ulcer in New York City during this century (from 1 to 1 to about 20 to 1).

This is slender evidence on which to base a general conclusion concerning the methods needed in mental illness. But at least past experience indicates that not much can be expected from 'more of the same' that is to say from extension of improved feeding and elimination of physical hazards. The variation in experience of different societies suggests that social institutions and behaviour contribute largely to the occurrence of psychological illness, and it seems reasonable to believe that it is to their modification we must look eventually for prevention and control.

Geriatric illness

The increased volume of disease and disability in late life is attributable mainly to the increase in population age. Assessment of the scope for different measures should take account of the following points.

The traditional methods have been much less successful than in younger age-groups, increased expectation of life during this century being at most a few years from middle and late life. Probably the most important reason for the refractory character of pathological conditions in this age-group is that at the end of reproductive life they are less likely to be eliminated by natural selection.

Nevertheless there is substantial scope for reduction of morbidity and mortality from conditions such as chronic bronchitis, coronary artery disease, and cancer of the lung by modification of the environment. However, the environment in question is largely the personal environment, whose control depends on changes in behaviour rather than external measures. Indeed in technologically advanced countries personal habits are probably now more important than other environmental influences; smoking, for example, has a more direct effect on the lungs than the residual amount of atmospheric pollution, and the individual's decision about what and how much he eats is more significant than the general availability of food.

Although lives of the elderly can often be prolonged by treatment, the increase in life expectation is inevitably small in comparison with that which has resulted from other methods in younger age-groups. Moreover the aged who survive as a result of treatment are not usually restored to full health but are in greater or lesser degree disabled. Hence a large and probably increasing proportion of the work for the elderly consists of prolonged care of the physically or mentally disabled.

THE MEDICAL TASK

In the preceding discussion it was concluded that the most important requirements for the health of living things are limitation of numbers and environmental measures; the environmental measures comprise provision of sufficient food, and protection from external hazards (such as predation, accidents, parasites, and—in the case of man—homicide) whose character varies considerably between different species and, to some extent, for the same species at different times. Human needs are essentially the same as those of other animals; what is different is the means of meeting them, since in man, because of ethical restraints control of reproduction must be learned rather than imposed.

These conclusions are consistent with interpretation of the

reasons for improvement of man's health. In Britain the major influences appear to have become effective in this order: increase in food supplies from the mid eighteenth century, hygienic measures from 1870, and limitation of numbers from about the same time. Effective prevention and treatment of disease in the individual were delayed until the second quarter of the twentieth century and have been less significant than any of the other major influences.

In the developing countries of the world today, the main requirement is for the traditional measures, although they need not be, and probably will not be, applied in the same order as in western Europe. Because of its cheapness, control of environmental hazards is preceding a general improvement in food supplies and standards of living and this change in timing has made limitation of numbers even more urgent than it would otherwise be.

In technologically advanced countries, the scope of the traditional measures is still far from being exhausted. Nevertheless the character of health problems has changed, and will increasingly change, from those which were predominant during man's evolution to the residual problems which remain. These are essentially congenital, psychiatric, and geriatric.

Within the foreseeable future—and with such complex issues it is of little use to attempt to look further—the solution of congenital problems will require particularly: identification and elimination by abortion of the abnormal embryo or foetus; improved obstetric care, to protect the mother and ensure the safe birth of the normal child; specific prevention and treatment of disease in the newborn, where this is possible; and care of children with residual disabilities (the mentally defective, the congenitally malformed, etc.) who have been neither identified during pregnancy nor effectively treated after birth. The last is likely to remain a large part of the medical task resulting from congenital disability.

The scope for different measures in the prevention, treatment, and care of mental illness remains an open question and what follows is no more than a personal opinion. With some notable exceptions in the case of specific forms of mental illness, the contribution of physical and chemical methods derived from the engineering approach will not be large. In time, however, it may be possible to make substantial advances by modification of ways of life through changes in social institutions and behaviour.

In middle and late life improvements in health can be expected from modification of personal behaviour, particularly in respect of habits which represent a profound departure from the conditions of life in which man evolved. But though such changes will reduce the volume of disease and disability in the elderly, it will still be large. Specific therapeutic measures are of value, but in late life can offer only a marginal increase in expectation of life. Moreover those who survive will often be left with residual disabilities, and the care of the disabled will remain a large part of the medical task in this age-group.

Taking account of both the traditional measures, and of additional methods already available in the foreseeable future, the various influences on which health depends may be classified as follows:

Modification of behaviour

(*a*) Control of reproduction, mainly in limitation of family size and possibly to a small extent in selective breeding.

(*b*) Changes in behaviour which prejudices the individual's own health (for example by smoking, lack of exercise, and excessive eating).

(*c*) Changes in behaviour which affects the health of others. They may concern a wide range of influences, from the mother's handling of her child and the relation between husband and wife to social behaviour and organization.

Since behaviour determines both the vital limitation of numbers and the control of personal habits which are crucial to health, even if no large assumptions are made about its contribution to the prevention of mental illness, it is probable that it includes the most important influences on human health.

Environmental measures

Although a distinction is usually made between provision of sufficient food and protection from physical hazards, they can be considered together as environmental measures. Their past and continuing importance has been sufficiently stressed and only one point need be added here: that changing conditions of life bring new hazards which require new methods of protection.

Prevention and treatment of disease in the individual

Some of the most successful applications of the engineering approach are in problems which should not arise, for example in treatment of road accidents and obesity. If such conditions are prevented by behavioural and environmental measures, the following are among the important uses which would remain.

(*a*) In pregnancy and childhood: identification and elimination by abortion of abnormal embryos, improved obstetric care, specific preventive and therapeutic measures in the newborn. It is probable that the engineering approach has its greatest potential usefulness in this period.

(*b*) In middle and late life: prevention, identification, and treatment of disease and disability. But while these services will increasingly engage the attention of the medical services, and will offer great scope for technology, it is questionable whether they can be expected to make a large contribution through prevention of disability and extension of life.

Care of the disabled

The size of the problem presented by the disabled will be determined by several things; for example by ability to identify and abort the abnormal foetus and by intervention to prolong the lives of the seriously disabled (as in the treatment of spina bifida). But with due regard for such uncertainties, even if all the measures referred to above were energetically applied, it can hardly be doubted that the number of disabled patients requiring prolonged care would still be very large. They are prominent among all three of the major residual classes: the congenitally disabled, the mentally ill, and the elderly.

This appraisal underlines the past and continuing importance to health of behavioural and environmental influences. It suggests that they are much more significant than specific measures of preventing and treating disease, which nevertheless are of great value in pregnancy and early childhood and, to a lesser extent, in late life. But the character of the residual problems which are now predominant in technologically advanced societies, suggests that in the foreseeable future large numbers of disabled patients will remain after the application of preventive and therapeutic measures. The care of such patients represents a substantial and increasing proportion of the medical task.

The conclusion to be drawn is, not that medicine should turn away from the engineering approach, but that the approach needs to be seen in perspective by recognition that the health of man, like that of other living things, depends primarily on methods directed to populations rather than to individuals. When these methods are applied effectively, the scope for specific preventive and therapeutic measures is greatly reduced except in respect of certain residual congenital, geriatric and, less certainly, psychiatric problems which characterize the medical task in technologically advanced societies. The usefulness of specific measures may prove to be greatest in prenatal life, particularly if it becomes possible to recognize and abort the seriously abnormal embryo.

Against this background it can be seen that the main requirement is to exploit fully the traditional environmental and behavioural methods, and if possible extend them in the control of mental illness. Since most serious diseases and disabilities are likely to prove relatively intractable if they cannot be prevented, the role of therapeutic medicine should be modified to include as the major commitment the concept of care. Such a change would carry important implications for medical science and service and should affect the content and orientation of medical education.

SUMMARY

Since the time of Kepler and Harvey, medical thought has been dominated by the belief that improvements in health must rely largely on an engineering approach, based on understanding of the structure and function of the body and of the disease processes which affect it. In fact man's health offers only limited scope for this approach. Past improvement has been due mainly to modification of behaviour and changes in the environment and it is to these same influences that we must look particularly for further advance. This interpretation does not overlook what is sometimes referred to as the pastoral role of the doctor; on the contrary, it underlines its significance, for since most major diseases and disabilities are either preventable or intractable, care rather than cure should be our concept of the main focus of personal medical attention.

These conclusions are derived from (*a*) interpretation of the improvement in health which has occurred since the eighteenth century, (*b*) appraisal of the major influences on the health of living things and of the ethical restraints on their application to man, and (*c*) assessment of the character of the residual health problems in technologically advanced countries.

REFERENCES

1. CROMBIE, A. C. (1966). 'The future of biology: the history of a program', *Federation Proc.* 25, no. 5, 1448–53.

2. McKEOWN, T., and RECORD, R. G. (1962). 'Reasons for the decline of mortality in England and Wales during the nineteenth century', *Popul. Stud.* 16, 94–122.

3. HART, P. D., and WRIGHT, G. P. (1939). *Tuberculosis and Social Conditions in England* (London: National Association for the Prevention of Tuberculosis).

4. RAZZELL, P. E. (1965). 'Population change in eighteenth century England. A reinterpretation', *Econ. Hist. Rev.*, second series, 18, 312–32.

5. DOWNIE, A. W. (1965). 'Comment on: "Edward Jenner: the history of a medical myth" by Razzell, P. E.', *Med. Hist.* 9, 223–5.

6. HELLEINER, K. F. (1957). 'The vital revolution reconsidered', *Can. J. Econ. pol. Sci.* 23, 1–9.

7. HUTCHINSON, J. (1966). 'Land and human populations', *Listener*, 1 Sept. 303–11.

8. Ernle, R. E. P. (1919). *English Farming Past and Present* (London : Longmans Green).

9. Andrewes, C. H. (1966). 'Viruses and evolution', *The Huxley Lecture* (University of Birmingham).

10. Wynne-Edwards, V. C. (1962). *Animal Dispersion in Relation to Social Behaviour* (Edinburgh : Oliver & Boyd).

11. Lack, D. (1966). *Population Studies of Birds* (Oxford : Clarendon Press).

Discussion

REASONS FOR IMPROVEMENT IN HEALTH

A general interpretation of reasons for improvement in human health undoubtedly presents difficulties. Some are philosophic in kind, for example the problem of defining what comprises improvement; one may be physically healthy and unhappy, or disabled and happy. There are several reasons for scientific difficulty, particularly uncertainty concerning the reliability of diagnoses before the late nineteenth century.

The problem is perhaps more tractable when fragmented, by separate consideration of the behaviour of individual diseases such as plague, typhus, typhoid, and cholera. A great deal of attention has been devoted rightly to tuberculosis, and the interpretations are in general accord with the one suggested in the preceding paper. Nevertheless the broader interpretation should not lose sight of the advances recently achieved by specific measures. They are illustrated by the treatment of tuberculosis since about 1948, immunization against diphtheria, and the prevention and treatment of rickets, a nutritional disease. It is only by separate and detailed analysis of this kind that it is possible to feel confident about the conclusions reached in a general interpretation.

In the USA a recent investigation has extended the detailed examination of reasons for the trend of mortality into the twentieth century. The conclusions are consistent with those reached in the earlier period (1); the most important influences have been food and hygiene.

Although the importance of improvements in nutrition has been recognized, its influence has not hitherto been dissociated from other features of a rising standard of living such as better housing and a safe water supply. The case for regarding improved food as a major influence on the decline of mortality in Britain in the eighteenth and early nineteenth centuries rests on evidence which is both direct and indirect: there were undoubtedly large increases in food supplies; a population which trebled between 1700 and 1850 was fed almost entirely on home-grown food; other explanations for a large decline in mortality (specific medical measures, advances in hygiene, or a fortuitous decline in mortality from infectious disease) cannot be substantiated; and an improvement in nutrition is the kind of influence which would be expected to have a profound effect on mortality in a population which was seriously undernourished. At the same time it should be recognized that the improvement in nutrition was not wholly due to advances in agriculture. Other important influences were better transportation which facilitated the distribution of food, a rising standard of living associated with the Industrial Revolution which increased the level of real wages, and advances in understanding of methods of keeping and preparing food. Without such influences the impact on health of improvements in agriculture would have been greatly reduced.

The preceding paper attached great importancce to the behavioural change which led to the decline of the birth-rate in the late nineteenth century, but concluded that the behavioural mechanisms which are considered by some writers (2) to have restricted the size of animal populations have had little relevance to man. Contemporary experience suggests that in general this is true; in developing countries there is no evidence of effective control of reproduction which keeps population size within the limits that can be supported by the available food. Nevertheless there are examples of such a mechanism in man, in Australian aboriginal populations whose growth appears to be controlled by such influences as infanticide, abortion, and complex intermarriage arrangements.

The importance attached to control of numbers in the preceding paper may be thought to imply a concept of optimum size of population. To be acceptable such a concept needs to be stated very explicitly, and to be supported by the evidence on which it is based. In general it is assumed that populations should be smaller, although there are econominc and social conditions under which a larger population may be desirable. These considerations should lead to caution in accepting a concept of optimum population size, although they are not inconsistent with the general conclusions concerning the significance of the decline of the birth-rate in Britain since about 1870. It can hardly be doubted that had the birth-rate remained unchanged the population of Britain would have trebled in the past century, and the prevention of this rate of growth made an outstanding contribution to the subsequent improvement in health.

RESIDUAL HEALTH PROBLEMS

In the discussion of residual health problems it was concluded that there is little prospect of reducing the incidence of serious disease and disability by contraception requiring identification of parents whose children are likely to be affected. The possibility of improving the human race by artificial selection of parents has also been discussed since the time of Galton. This approach is not in tune with contemporary opinion, for even if the technical difficulties could be overcome, there would remain strong ethical objections to the concept of selective breeding in man. In *The Golden Fleece*, Robert Graves refers to an island on which there were many small boys whose shortness of temper and sturdiness of frame identified them as the offspring of Achilles. This illustrates one of the problems which would confront the controllers of human breeding, that it would be impossible to anticipate the consequences of selection for characters which are desired on characters which are unwanted.

Ideas concerning the nature and possible control of mental illness are inevitably controversial. Here it may be important to distinguish clearly between neurotic and psychotic illness. The incidence of the former is extremely variable and the influences, presumably environmental, which are mainly responsible are largely unknown. The incidence of psychotic illness, on the other hand, appears to be remarkably constant and it has many features of organic disease which may well prove susceptible to control by what has been referred to as the engineering approach.

In the examination of reasons for improvement in health attention has understandably focused on mortality, in respect of which data are available over a considerable period from national sources. However, it must not be forgotten that there is also a large volume of morbidity which is responsible for much distress and may lead to prolonged disability. An appraisal of residual health problems should, so far as possible, take account of it.

Finally it should be recognized that the residual health problems described are those of advanced societies and the picture is very different in developing countries. Here the order of events in the West has been changed; medicine is outstripping the development of agriculture and industry, because effective and economical environmental measures such as spraying are causing a decline of mortality from infectious disease which is far in advance of a rising standard of living and control of population growth. Although the point is theoretical, the health and welfare of these countries might be better if the major influences had developed along eighteenth-century rather than twentieth-century lines. Such issues are of course economic and political as well as medical, but medicine can contribute by identifying the major influences on health and by clarifying the consequences of their modification.

THE MEDICAL TASK

The preceding discussion rightly attributes great importance to modification of behaviour, particularly in relation to limitation of popular growth. Interest in this influence is relatively new for medicine, which traditionally has been concerned to preserve life rather than to restrict numbers. Indeed the main reasons for limitation of family size have been social and economic rather than medical; it is the concern of parents for their own and their children's welfare rather than their health that leads them to decide to have fewer children. However, attention is beginning to be drawn to the significance of numbers of offspring to health, for example by the Family Planning movement in relating their programmes to the health of mother and child.

The control of numbers presents medicine with a dilemma, since there are only three effective methods: to kill people; to allow them to die; and to practise birth control. The first method is unacceptable, the second is controversial, and only the third is really practicable. Unfortunately this subject is surrounded by social and religious prejudices or principles, the precise designation being determined largely by the individual's personal viewpoint. However, the problem is urgent and inescapable, and it must be faced, first by doctors and later by society as a whole.

There is little likelihood of dispute about the continued importance of environmental influences. Indeed the evidence concerning them is being extended, for example in the demonstration of an inverse relationship between the level of calcium in water supplies and the manifestation of cardiovascular disease. If substantiated, this evidence might lead to environmental measures which could have a profound effect on this common cause of mortality.

It should, of course, be recognized that in many circumstances environmental and behavioural influences are intimately related. For example in developing countries it will be difficult to persuade people to use a safe water supply if it is available only at a considerable distance. A disease such as bilharzia might be prevented either by elimination of the infection or by teaching people not to go into infected water. And in the problem of birth control, behavioural patterns are almost inseparable from economic and other considerations. In this context it is worth recalling that education is not merely knowing more but is behaving differently.

The present is clearly a period of major change in medicine, change brought about by the pressure of society, and by changes in training programmes, delivery systems, and—in the USA—in finance of medical services. In such circumstances the role of medicine needs to be redefined, and it is probable that the conceptual model provided by the engineering approach will need to be enlarged.

REFERENCES

1. McKeown, T., and Record, R. G. (1962). 'Reasons for the decline of mortality in England and Wales during the nineteenth century', *Popul. Stud.* 16, 94–122.

2. Wynne-Edwards, V. C. (1962). *Animal Dispersion in Relation to Social Behaviour* (Edinburgh : Oliver and Boyd).

3

HISTORICAL TRENDS AND FUTURE PROSPECTS IN PUBLIC HEALTH

GEORGE ROSEN

Historical trends and future prospects in public health

Public health as an area of social activity owes its existence basically to the biosocial nature of man. As biological organisms, human beings are subject to fundamental needs such as alimentation and excretion, and exist by virtue of vital processes whose varying functional consequences and manifestations are summed up in concepts of health and disease. Throughout history, men living in large or small social units have had to reckon in some way with consequences of these facts for the well-being of the group.

The ways in which this has been done have been determined or at least strongly influenced by the nature and the social organization of the society or group, and by the knowledge and the technical means available to it. Human beings live in society as members of social groups. Their relations to their fellows in such groups can be conceived as social articulations or systems which in more permanent form can become social institutions. Taken together, these systems make up the social structure, the social organization of society.

In living together, men encounter problems relating to health which affect individuals and groups. All societies have some arrangement to deal with such problems. Such an arrangement or organization may have to deal with the control of transmissible disease, the provision of water and food of good quality and in sufficient supply, the cleaning of the physical environment, the provision of medical care, and the relief of disability and destitution. How such organizations are constituted, and how they carry out their tasks, are determined by influences and factors deriving from various areas of community life. Considered as social functions, the activities of the organizations that deal with group health problems are interlocked in varying degree with other elements in the structure of society, for example, with government, economic organization, religious institutions, the family, and the value system associated with them. Thus, understanding the nature and cause of disease can provide a basis for dealing with its occurrence and the needs of affected individuals. Yet the application of such knowledge more often than not depends less on the urgency of the health problem than on political, economic, ideological, and cultural factors. Current examples are obvious in efforts to deal with pollution of air and water, to reduce motor-vehicle accidents, to provide sex education in schools, or to deal with problems of malnutrition. The existence of health problems does not mean that attention will be directed to them, nor does accretion and availability of knowledge assure application. As William H. Welch noted in 1925, 'the health field has a woefully ineffective distribution service as compared with its marvelously effective production service in the laboratories of the world. We know how to do a lot of things which we won't do or do on a wretchedly small scale' (1).

Community action to deal with matters of health occurs in one form or another from the earliest cultures right up to the present in the varied regions and countries of the world. However, the instrumental expressions of such action have varied greatly, changing with altered social conditions, and in turn creating situations requiring other forms of social action. This is the history of public health. By investigating this history it is possible to understand forces and trends that have led to problems of our own time, and perhaps to grasp the possibilities for further change.

In the context of this conference it would be more useful not to review the history of public health, but rather to turn attention to the emergence of new forms of community health action in Great Britain and the United States in the nineteenth century, and to examine how these developments have led to the present. Organized public health agencies, modern style, were created to deal with the occurrence of epidemics and the prevalence of endemic disease in the urban centres of the early industrial society. They developed in response to social needs within a definite context resulting from the convergence of public and private factors. A leading aspect of the question of how to organize life in an increasingly urban and industrial society was the protection of the community's health. The problem of the public health was inherent in the new industrial civilization. The process that created the market economy, the factory, and the modern urban centre also brought into being the health problems that made necessary new means of health protection.

The health situation in the British cities and towns, as well as in their American counterparts during the earlier ninteenth century was a consequence of their evolution. The rapid aggregation of people in limited spaces was bound to produce stresses and strains and to create problems. The health of a population depends on many factors, among which a high place must be given to the standard of living, including as it does nutrition, housing, clothing, and medical care. What happened in the British and American cities in the earlier nineteenth century was that the pressures of industrialization and economic individualism, particularly when applied to people, many of whom were just becoming urbanized, created a state of cultural shock and depressed living standards for many to such a degree as to create a sense of apprehension, anxiety, and dismay in those about them (2–7).

The fear and dismay aroused by these developments had two major and related aspects. One was a reaction to the different way of life of the workers and the poor, a sense that there was something unknown, mysterious and dangerous about the lower orders of society, that the alleys and the rookeries in which they lived were rife with all kinds of evil and morbidity.

These attitudes were not limited to the British; they were shared with the French, the Americans, and the Germans. After all it was Eugène Sue who first wrote *Les Mystères de Paris* in 1843, and Charles Loring Brace, who produced *The Dangerous Classes of New York* in 1872, two popular expressions of these attitudes. The culture of poverty, to use a current phrase, in its values, experience and life style denied in large measure all that the middle class officially espoused and held dear. As Dickens put it specifically in terms of education, the school

> was childish and innocent. . . . Young women old in the vices of the commonest and worst life, were expected to profess themselves enthralled by the good child's book, the Adventures of Little Margery, who resided in the village cottage by the mill . . . who plaited straw and delivered the dreariest orations to all comers, at all sorts of unseasonable times (8).

Underlying the feelings and attitudes aroused by this cultural and psychological confrontation was the concern aroused by specific urban problems, such as overcrowding, destitution, crime, alcoholism, prostitution, illegitimacy, and disease which seemed to be inextricably intertwined. Death and disease seemed to lurk in the houses and haunts of the poor ready to emerge as epidemics to threaten the health and life of their betters. Thus, exploration of the dark alleys of poverty in the ninteenth-century city went hand in hand with horrified and fascinated investigation of disease, particularly of the aspects which aroused public opinion through fear or because they seemed to lead to evil consequences of such magnitude that they could not be sustained. Various legislative enactments concerned with the public health were the result of reactions to revealed abuses and threats. The Public Health Act of 1848 was due as much to the threat of cholera as it was to the revelations and exhortations of crusading reformers. Similarly, the cholera epidemic of 1853 led to the Act of 1855 which consolidated and amended the Nuisances Removal and Disease Prevention Acts, and obliged local authorities to take action on sanitary matters. This was true as well of the Arsenic Act of 1857 and the 1860 Act for Preventing the Adulteration of Articles of Food and Drink, and of the Act creating the Metropolitan Board of Health in New York in 1866.

Whatever the motivation, action to deal with health problems had to be taken in terms of available knowledge, and it was precisely on this point that medical science was deficient. Nevertheless, action was taken along certain lines. Vaccination reduced the incidence of smallpox. The ravages of enteric infections were diminished by the drive for sanitation of the environment through the removal of filth and excrement, and the provision of clean water. For the most part, however, improvement in the health status of the urban population was achieved essentially by improvement in the standards of living of the poorer and most numerous classes of the community.

The English experience with typhus fever illustrates this development. After 1869, when typhus fever began to be tabulated separately in the Registrar-General's Reports, it ceased to be epidemic, leading to an almost continuous decline in the number of fatal attacks. In 1869, there were 4,281 typhus deaths in England; by 1885 the number had dropped to 318. The corresponding rates per thousand living were 0·19 and 0·01. Individual cities reflected the general trend. London, for example, had 716 typhus deaths in 1869 and only 28 in 1885; during this period the death rate per thousand living for typhus declined from 0·23 to 0·01. Typhus fever did not totally disappear in Britain during the nineteenth century, but it no longer had any serious epidemiologic importance after 1900 (9–11). By 1906, three years before Charles Nicolle's discovery that the body louse transmitted typhus, the annual report of the London County Council stated that there were no more deaths from the disease that year.

How had this change come about even though the cause of typhus remained unknown? These trends undoubtedly reflect in large measure the impact of the sanitary reform movement during the ninteenth century. 'The discovery of the laws of public health', the Registrar-General noted in 1871, 'the determination of the conditions of cleanliness, manners, food, exercise, isolation, medicine most favourable to life in one city, in one country, is a boon to every city, to every country, for all can profit by the experience' (12). In the eyes of the sanitary reformers, a clean city was bound to be a healthy city. Acting on this premise, they undertook to clean up the physical environment, to improve housing, to provide pure water in adequate supply, and unadulterated food on a regular basis, in short, to provide decent living conditions.

It had long been noted that the occurrence and prevalence of typhus were closely related to the socio-economic circumstances of its victims. Typhus fever was found to be closely associated with poverty, destitution, poor housing, overcrowding, and poor personal hygiene; and was not inaccurately called the poor man's disease. It was not a characteristic health problem of the middle and upper classes of nineteenth-century Britain, except for those such as physicians, nurses, the clergy, and others whose occupations brought them into contact with the sick, the dead, or their surroundings. Most municipalities throughout the nineteenth century never even came within sight of overtaking problems of community hygiene and health. Nevertheless, enough positive change did take place to yield ascertainable benefits. Slum clearance, regulation of lodging-houses, provision of public baths and wash-houses, increased use of cotton clothing, particularly underwear, and consequent improvement in personal cleanliness played their part in reducing the prevalence of typhus fever. Slum clearance tended to disperse the workers to newer districts where they could live without excessive crowding because new means of transportation also became available. Real wages generally rose during the second half of the nineteenth century and living costs fell in Britain, particularly as cheap imported foodstuffs became more available. As Charles Creighton observed in 1884, 'food has been for a long time cheap and wages good. . . . So long as our cheap supplies of food, fuel and clothing are uninterrupted, there is small chance of typhus or relapsing fever' (11).

Seen in retrospect such historical developments as the decline of typhus seem clear and straight, but the process from which they are abstracted was not so smooth. What looks like a steady even advance over several decades is seen under closer scrutiny to consist of hesitant piecemeal changes, *ad hoc* expedients, and compromises resulting from bitterly waged campaigns against specific evils. Actions were taken by urban communities, or were forced upon them, to remedy specific and glaring sanitary deficiencies without necessarily considering how far these were related to other problems. Nevertheless, the thread of continuity it not an illusion, an artifact of the historian. It is a reality derived from the circumstances that throughout most of the nineteenth century and into the twentieth century health workers confronted substantially similar problems. Undesirable conditions and situations like those uncovered in urban communities by the classic investigations of the 1830s and 1840s were still being explored in the 1880s and 1890s (13). Even the reasons for these conditions were not dissimilar.

Charles Booth, who surveyed the working-class districts of London from 1889 to 1902, felt that the general level of living had improved. Yet Booth's investigations in London and Rowntree's study of York in 1899 showed that a substantial portion of the labouring population was living on incomes beneath a subsistence level (14–15). The more thoroughly the condition of the poorer classes in the community was investigated, the more unsatisfactory their health and social situation was found to be. Malnutrition was rife and the health and physical fitness of the more poorly paid members of the working class was defective. Maternal mortality was high. While infant mortality had declined, the condition of children attending school as well as that of pre-school children was found to be extremely poor (16–18).

Similar evils were present in the great cities of the United States. Slum areas were not new in American cities. Indeed, the health problems presented by these phenomena in the mid nineteenth century had led to the creation of the first modern health departments (19). At the end of the nineteenth century, however, this problem became extremely acute. Industrial expansion, urban growth, and a new flood of immigration all coincided to produce congested areas in which thousands of people huddled in unbelievably inadequate housing deprived of some of the most elementary requirements of civilized life. Poverty, malnutrition, disease, and vice were widespread. The descriptions by Jacob Riis of slum conditions in New York equalled, if they did not surpass, the conditions depicted by Booth and Rowntree in England (20–2).

Nevertheless, the sheer magnitude of these problems no longer appeared quite so overwhelming. Factual knowledge of such conditions, and the conscience and drive to do something about them, combined with more knowledge as to disease causation led officials and concerned citizens to redress such shortcomings. When it was accepted in the nineteenth century that communicable diseases (epidemic and endemic) were related to filthy environmental conditions (water supply, sewerage, food supply), the appropriate solution appeared to be a preventive programme applying engineering knowledge and techniques in a consistent manner. During this period, the later nineteenth century, the sanitation of the environment to control communicable diseases and to improve living conditions comprised the practice of public health, with the sanitary engineer and the physician as the chief figures in the field. The provision of personal health services (medical care) concerned public health only in so far as individuals were affected by such communicable diseases. Moreover, the indigent were the responsibility of the poor law authorities and the workhouse infirmaries (23–4).

Public health authorities operated within administrative structures newly created to deal with the urgent problems of sanitary reform. Examples are the General Board of Health in England (1848) and the New York Metropolitan Board of Health (1866).

'How quaint the ways of Paradox!' observed Sir William Gilbert and this comment is certainly applicable to the role of medicine in the development of public health action. Analysis of the sanitary reform movement in England and the United States indicates that medicine played a secondary role in the process. The impulse to sanitary reform did not come mainly from the medical profession, even though physicians played an important part in calling attention to the community problems of ill-health and their presumed causes. Furthermore, medicine had little solid knowledge to contribute toward a solution of the major problem, the origin and spread of various diseases. It is indeed noteworthy that the programme of the sanitary reformers was to a large extent based on erroneous theories, and while they advocated appropriate solutions it was chiefly for the wrong reasons. Broadly speaking, what happened was that the founders of modern public health established institutional forms to carry out programmes which appeared reasonable in terms of what they thought they knew, and in terms of what the community through its dominant groups was prepared to accept. These institutions were to be available later, at the end of the nineteenth century and in the twentieth century, to put into practice more accurate medical and biological knowledge.

Concurrently, knowledge was accumulating that pointed to an animate contagion as the cause of infectious disease. The work of Louis Pasteur and Robert Koch marked the beginning of the golden age of bacteriology and immunology. By the end of the nineteenth century, some of the pertinent questions concerning communicable diseases and their prevention had been answered, and it became possible for this knowledge to be applied in public health programmes. The first decade of the twentieth century had a solid basis for the control of a number of infectious diseases, and throughout succeeding decades up to the present advances along this line have continued.

Many important communicable diseases had begun to wane before the full effects of the bacteriological discoveries made themselves felt. Beginning about 1870, there was a continuing downward trend in mortality due to a decline in the frequency of certain diseases, chiefly smallpox, typhoid and typhus fevers, and tuberculosis (10, 23–7). In the United States those great epidemic terrors, cholera and yellow fever, disappeared, never to return, before the specific causes of these infections were discovered and before exact knowledge of their transmission became known. These trends were roughly the same in the technologically advanced areas, particularly the municipalities, of Western Europe and America, and were reinforced by the application of bacteriological, immunological, and eventually chemotherapeutic knowledge.

Children and young adults were the chief beneficiaries from

the victories won in the battle against communicable diseases. The degree of benefit obtained from measures for the improvement of water and milk is clearly shown by the trend in infant mortality in New York City. In 1885 the infant death-rate was 273 per thousand live-birth; by 1915 it had dropped sharply to 94 per thousand (28–9). This great gain in child life has had a considerable impact on the development of community health problems and action over the past fifty years. Not only were many lives saved but also more infants grew up to adulthood. There is no doubt that the decline in the mortality of younger age-groups has been an important element in the appearance of a larger number of old people in the United States, Great Britain, and other economically advanced countries.

Alongside these trends, during the decades preceding the First World War, a shift was beginning to take place in the concept and orientation of public health, a shift of attention from the environment to the individual. As health authorities and others became aware of noxious influences other than those emanating from the physical environment, as activities in connection with maternal and child health, industrial hygiene, nutrition, tuberculosis, venereal disease, and mental ill-health developed, the scope of public health expanded. As new areas of concern became part of public health, new programmes developed and new personnel were trained to execute them (30–1). Moreover, it is essential to keep in mind that much of this development of public health in official agencies took place because no other institution was readily available to handle at least in some degree the consequences of poverty and ill-health which were so widespread in Britain and the United States at the end of the nineteenth century and during the early decades of the present century. 'In the homes of the poor', Edward T. Devine wrote in 1910, 'we find the dire consequences of death and disease, of unemployment and underemployment, of overwork and nervous strain, of dark and ill ventilated and overcrowded rooms; of undernourishment and exposure and poisoned food, of ignorance and maladjustment' (32).

For the most part the problems with which public health was

concerned affected specific groups of the population, most of which were also poor. Proper sewerage and clean water supplies were of service to the entire community and prevented diseases such as typhoid fever which might attack members of any social class. However, it was clear that a low standard of living had a deleterious effect on nutritional status, infant and child health, tuberculosis, venereal disease, occupational health, and on the quality and availability of medical care. Many of the sick poor were not in a position to obtain medical care through private practitioners, and flocked to the out-patient departments and wards of the voluntary hospitals. As early as 1846, Lord Ashley's Committee on Medical Poor Relief proposed the establishment of a system of public dispensaries to be financed through public as well as private contributions (33). No action was taken on these proposals; but important personal health and welfare services, such as maternity and child care, home nursing and ambulance service, were developed by local authorities. Some authorities also administered hospitals, especially for such diseases as tuberculosis.

At the same time paralleling these developments were the efforts to provide some degree of security against the hardships of unemployment, ill-health, old age, and premature death. The Royal Commission appointed in 1905 to examine the problem of the Poor Law in all its aspects provided the point of departure for future developments. Despite a large measure of agreement on the basic issues, the Commissioners differed on the means to deal with them and issued a Majority and a Minority Report, each taking a profoundly different approach (34–5). The Minority Report, largely the work of Beatrice Webb, proposed a unified state medical service, to combine the Poor Law medical services with those provided by public health authorities, the whole to be administered by a national health department as part of a social security system. The Majority Report proposed a less radical, more piecemeal approach. They retained the Poor Law, but introduced various measures such as unemployment insurance and health insurance to cushion the hardships inherent in the untrammelled operation of the industrial system.

These proposals were enacted in 1911 as 'An Act to provide for Insurance against Loss of Health and for the Prevention and Care of Sickness, and for Insurance against Unemployment and for purposes incidental thereto.' Then in 1919 another recommendation of the Poor Law Commission became a reality with the establishment of the Ministry of Health, which took over the health functions of the Local Government Board, the health insurance organization, the health and medical inspection duties of the Ministry of Education, as well as other matters relating to health such as epidemics, sanitation, and housing.

Although these measures provided a basis for an integrated health service, the opportunities for integrating preventive and curative services was disregarded in 1911 and 1919. Similarly, the advice of the Royal Commission on National Health Insurance of 1926 in the same direction was ignored. Between 1920 and 1939, however, a number of notable studies and reports on health policy and the provision of health services were made. In 1920, the Dawson Committee, a consultative council to the Ministry of Health, recommended the creation of a comprehensive health service which would provide preventive and curative care through a national system of health centres in two categories. One group would provide primary care through general physicians, dentists, nurses, midwives, and others; the other would provide specialist and consultant services, and both would be mutually dependent. Mention might also be made of the Sankey Report, and the PEP Report, both issued in 1937 and both indicating a need for change and improvement in the organization and delivery of health services (36–9). The coming of the Second World War thrust upon Britain the need for planning, not least in health. There was considerable evidence of the existence of a vast amount of avoidable ill-health, in part a result of the great depression of the 1930s, and in part a legacy of earlier generations (40–3). At the same time many health institutions, specifically the hospitals, were in dire straits. Studies by independent investigators had left no doubt that the organization of the hospitals lagged behind public needs and was failing to bring the advances of medical knowledge adequately within the reach of the people (44). There was a demonstrated need for the rationalization and co-ordination of services and facilities that had been developed to deal with specific problems and specific groups of the population and with little relationship to each other. Moreover, all too often the efficiency of the service or the facility was related to the resources of the local authority or the voluntary agency charged with administrative responsibility.

The exigencies of the war burst through the barriers of special interests, party politics, hesitation, and inertia, and set in motion a process of change and reform that had been long overdue. To create an Emergency Medical Service leaders in medicine and public health worked together with government officials, and dealt with problems of policy and organization on a national basis (45). Many of these trends and currents of thought were brought together in 1942 when the Beveridge Report on *Social Insurance and Allied Services* pointed out that social security cannot be fully provided unless health needs are cared for along comprehensive lines (46). Some form of comprehensive health service was inevitable as a major step of health and social policy, and in February 1944 there appeared a White Paper on *A National Health Service* (39). The central feature of the proposals contained in it was the joint health authority, or area health board, with broad comprehensive functions for planning, organization, and administration.

Nevertheless, when the NHS was created by the Act of 1946, this feature and the principles underlying it were not followed, the opportunity to fashion an integrated health service was disregarded, and a trend toward the provision of more comprehensive health services under local government was reversed. This development occurred despite the fact that medical officers of health in local units had successfully demonstrated during the war years (1939–45) their ability to organize and administer health services in difficult and complex situations, a fact emphasized by the Chief Medical Officer to the Ministry of Health in his report of 1946 (47). The basic reason for avoiding an integrated service based on local health authorities was not because it was not feasible, but rather because it was impolitic. Hospitals and physicians were opposed to control by local authorities, and the national government could not ignore political realities (37, 48). These included not only the pressures of the medical profession and allied health groups, but also the outmoded and inadequate structure of local government (49). As a result, local government lost its potentially dominating role in the health services, and the NHS emerged divided into three parts like Gaul: a hospital and specialist service; a general physician, dental, pharmaceutical, and optical service; and a local health authority service. The functions left to the local health units under the NHS, after the loss of hospitals, comprised chiefly personal preventive services and certain aspects of domiciliary care in illness (maternal and child care, domiciliary midwifery, health visiting, home nursing, home help service, vaccination and immunization, aftercare of discharged hospital patients, mental health and welfare). Two new functions that were added were ambulance service and health centre administration. The latter has potentially the greatest significance for the future of public health, but as yet its potential remains unrealized.

In part, this situation was also a consequence of the very success of public health in earlier decades. When communicable diseases were everyday problems for communities, families, and individuals, action by health agencies to deal with such potential threats and actual perils was in the centre of public interest. Indeed, for many public health became identified with combatting communicable diseases, with microbe hunting, to such an extent that when most of the widely prevalent microbial conditions had been brought under control, public health found itself in a kind of limbo. After all there is little drama in keeping environmental and community conditions under control so that health threats will not develop. At the same time, the very success of public health in controlling infectious diseases led to the appearance of new problems for which solutions do not as yet exist. As a result of increased life expectancy at birth, larger numbers of people live longer. In consequence, among the problems that confront us today are the control of the much less remediable degenerative or chronic diseases: cancer, cardiovascular-renal conditions, diabetes mellitus, arthritis, musculoskeletal conditions, and mental changes associated with ageing. At the same time, the changing scope of public health has broadened to include other elements and situations that may adversely effect the physical and psychological well-being of the people, among them such problems as accident prevention, mental health, as well as renewed emphasis on the control of the physical environment. With an expanding and changing industrial technology have come environmental alterations of increasing complexity and danger. The once-dominant problems of bacterially contaminated air, water, and food have now been replaced to a very considerable degree by chemical pollution and problems of solid waste disposal. It is not necessary to go into detail, for the general situation is similar both in Great Britain and the United States, even though in the latter the organizational and political problems are different (50).

Changes in the age structure and morbidity patterns of countries such as Great Britain and the United States, the growth of scientific medicine, the greater availability of disposable income and a rising standard of living among large groups of people have led to greater demands for health care and higher levels of expectation concerning the health which a person might enjoy and the services and facilities necessary to provide care. These developments have given greater prominence and weight to institutions such as hospitals, where medical manpower and equipment are centralized, and to the industries that supply them (drugs, hospital supplies and equipment). In short, the place of public health cannot be understood in isolation from these developments (24). It is against the background sketched above that one must view the current situation and future prospects of public health.

On the one hand, there is a continuing tendency to diminish the current activities of the local health authority or to remove them altogether to other agencies. Recent evidence of this trend may be found in the suggestion of the Ministry of Health to transfer ambulance service to regional hospital boards, and in the proposal of the Seebohm Report to remove social services from local health departments. If the latter proposal should be accepted it would 'remove half [the] staff and a substantial part of their budget, contacts, and interests. Moreover, our proposals would involve loss of the services for the social care of the mentally ill which has been one of the main growing points of local authority health departments.' Indeed, 'the critical question is whether the local authority health and school department which remains after our proposed changes could be a viable working unit' (51). Obviously a question to be answered only in the spirit of the Walrus and the Carpenter. For the present at least the fate of the local health department and the future shape of public health remain unclear, but one fact is evident. British public health in the future will not be what it has been.

A similar trend is observable in the United States, although the process of dismantling health departments has not yet advanced as far as it apparently has in Great Britain. Nevertheless, there are indications that the ultimate consequence may be the same unless attention is given to the place and the role of public health in the restructuring of health services now going on in the United States. Examples are the separation of mental health activites in numerous instances from health agencies, the removal of environmental control programmes from health departments to other units of government, as well as the ambiguous and not very effective role of public health in dealing with the organization and delivery of personal health services, a major problem of community health (52). A sense of unease has been apparent in American public health for some two decades. A major theme of the annual meeting of the American Public Health Association in 1957 was, 'Is public health in tune with the times?' Yet it was not until the mid 1960s that the need to face the problem of the declining role of public health was considered seriously enough to take positive action.

In part, this has been a result of an ambivalent attitude to political action. Departments of public health are creatures of government, and as such the administrators and technical experts who run them are aware of their vulnerability to political attack. Furthermore, in reaction to the incompetence fostered by political patronage in public health agencies earlier in the century, American public health developed an 'apolitical' stance coupled with an ideology insisting on the elimination of politics from public health work and the elevation of such activities to a professional plane. Public health programmes should be judged on the basis of objective, standardized criteria and should not be subjected to arbitrary, individual opinions. Health workers should be employed on the basis of competence and merit, not because of connections or political pay-offs (53). To a very considerable extent these aims have been achieved, but this success has also had unanticipated consequences. As American public health became professionalized, it also tended to become bureaucratic and to insist on well-defined areas of competence for which special training was required. Furthermore, professionalization tended to turn many public health people to what were considered pursuits more appropriate for a professional group, for example, research and demonstration, and away from public controversy and political battles.

To these trends and tendencies must be added a lack of clarity and general agreement on objectives, and consequently an absence of realistic and specific programmes with which to achieve theoretically desirable objectives. Underlying this situation was undoubtedly the circumstance that despite numerous proposals and legislative enactments, there were no national guidelines for the development of health services until the publication in 1945 of Haven Emerson's *Local Health Units for the Nation*. The Emerson report is an important document in the development of American public health, but despite the activities which it generated it marked the end of an era. It was the logical outcome of the process initiated around 1910 to develop more effective local health services based on the county as a political and administrative unit. Nevertheless, the usefulness of the Emerson report and the patterns of community health service which it proposed were quite limited.

To understand this judgement it is necessary to appreciate the setting in which the report appeared. During the decades preceding the Second World War a number of important, even basic forces and trends had been instigating changes in economic and political organization, social institutions and habits, codes of behaviour, and value systems. Furthermore, some forty years ago it was already apparent that there were strikingly unequal rates of change in various sectors of our society. Some were altering rapidly, while others were lagging by comparison. Even then it was becoming evident that these unequal rates of change in different areas of social life were creating points of tension and zones of danger. One of these was that scientific discovery and technologic innovation were outstripping the development of organization for their most effective utilization. Since then, this question has remained a major social and health problem—how to organize personal health services so that the established results of scientific research can be utilized without undue delay and in appropriate forms to benefit those who need health care.

Moreover, this problem has been complicated even more during this period by dramatic demographic changes. Not only did the population of the United States increase greatly in number, but it also remained highly mobile, moving from village to city to suburb, and from one part of the country to another. The impact of these changes was clearly not envisaged by Emerson and his colleagues when they set up the doctrine of the county health unit and its basic services. Against this background, as well as that of the other developments sketched above, the conviction has grown that today's health and medical science offered much more than most people got, that the patterns of community health service set forth in 1945 were no longer adequate to deal with current problems. At the same time, however, one must note that the United States still has no national health policy and this has had an important influence on public health.

Efforts have been made to develop such a policy through the creation of a National Commission on Community Health Services in 1962 sponsored by the American Public Health Association and the National Health Council. From the final report of the Commission, *Health is a Community Affair* (1966), it is clear that there has been a highly significant change in the concept of public health responsibility. The sharp lines of responsibility that once characterized the activities of official public health agencies have been broken down, specifically with respect to the distinction between prevention and cure, and the need for a single system of care for the provision of personal health services.

Slowly the United States has begun to move toward a national health policy and a unified system to provide health care to all. Medicare, Medicaid, OEO Neighborhood Health Centers, Community Mental Health Centers—all represent some effort in this direction, as do the two Federally sponsored efforts at reorganizing and rationalizing the health care delivery system, that is, Regional Medical Programs and Comprehensive Health Planning. But to paraphrase Galileo, while it does move, we still have a long way to go. Regional Medical Programs and Comprehensive Health Planning can only be described as embryonic and all the other programmes have their troubles. But at least a beginning has been made and some benchmarks established.

FUTURE PROSPECTS

It is obviously not possible to give a detailed blueprint of things to come. There are, however, several points to be considered, and we may do so by using a statement made in 1951 by an international group of experts under the sponsorship of the World Health Organization.

> Modern public health [they said] has been developed during the last hundred years from primarily a legislative and police function to an applied science, which constitutes an important and integral part of social and economic evolution. The techniques used in health administration have consequently been changed to emphasize positive measures in planning and organizing the modern health services on a community basis, in order to create a healthy environment for the people, and in educating the public for active participation in health work (54).

The operational words in this statement are planning and organization. Great Britain and the United States face situations that require both functions. In both countries there is a need for an integrated system of comprehensive health services based on local administrative units. Although the two countries are at different levels of socio-medical development, both require planning: To plan for health requires health intelligence. According to Evang what is needed is

> careful, long-term planning based on epidemiological research instead of swiftly improvised solutions, minute weighing of priorities in relation to available resources, coordination to avoid overlapping and duplication of effort, and analysis of methods and assessment of results. And finally, more important than anything else, imagination and bold initiative to meet the new health problems which the rapid changes in human environment produce, and old ones which have not been solved ... (55).

Yet apparently in Britain 'little use is made of modern epidemiology to provide an intelligence system relevant to local needs in health and health services' (51, 56).

Health intelligence is meaningful, however, only if it is applied. This requires organization and administration, skills which are available among public health workers, and which can be applied most fruitfully and effectively within a community setting. Leadership and organization in the promotion of health, in preventive medicine, in calling attention to health problems have all been functions of public health in the past, and can be in the future. The future of public health is in the development of a community health service. The achievement of this goal requires clarity and agreement on objectives of action, leadership by those in public health, and recognition of the need to develop coalitions with interested groups and to develop political support to achieve the goals set forth. For example in 1969 at its annual meeting the Governing Council of the American Public Health Association set out 'to provide leadership in formulating national policies with respect to personal and environmental health services'.

In conclusion, whatever forms of organization, administration, and financing are developed, certain functions must be performed in the interest of national and community health: health intelligence, control of disease (communicable and chronic), care of mothers and children, health administration, environmental health control, health education and information, laboratory services and others. This does not mean that the community health service has to undertake all types of service involved in these functions. But it should be in a position to check standards of quality and performance and to provide leadership in improving conditions. This has been the role of public health in the past and it will continue to do so in the future.

REFERENCES

1. WELCH, WILLIAM H. (1925). *State Charities Aid Association News* (Dec.), 14, 2.

2. KAY, J. P. (1832). *The Moral and Physical Condition of the Working Classes Employed in the Cotton Manufacture in Manchester* (London: James Ridgway), p. 19.

3. FELKIN, W. (1839). 'Moral statistics of a district near Gray's Inn', *Jl statist. Soc. Lond.* 1, 541–2.

4. FRIPP, C. BOWLES (1839). 'Report of an inquiry into the condition of the working classes of the city of Bristol', ibid. 2, 368–75.

5. HANEY, R. A. (1840). *State of the Poor Classes in Great Towns. Substance of a Speech in the House of Commons, Feb. 4, 1840, on Moving for a Committee to Consider the Causes of Discontent* (London: Longman & Co.).

6. SYKES, M. A., GUY, W. A., and NEISON, F. G. P. (1848). 'Report of a Committee of the Council of the Statistical Society of London . . . to investigate the state of the inhabitants and their dwellings in Church Lane, St. Giles's', *Jl statist. Soc. Lond.* 11, 1–18.

7. HOLE, JAMES (1866). *The Homes of the Working Classes* (London: Longmans, Green & Co.), pp. 5–6.

8. DICKENS, CHARLES (1865). *Our Mutual Friend* (London: Oxford University Press, 1952), p. 215.

9. JENNER, WILLIAM (1893). *Lectures and Essays on Fevers and Diptheria* (London), Preface.

10. THORNE, THORNE R. (1888). *The Progress of Preventive Medicine during the Victorian Era, 1837–1887* (London: Shaw & Sons), pp. 5–14, 17–22, 24.

11. CREIGHTON, CHARLES (1894). *A History of Epidemics in Britain*, 2 vols. (Cambridge University Press), vol. ii, pp. 209–19.

12. JEPHSON, HENRY (1907). *The Sanitary Evolution of London* (Brooklyn, N.Y.: A. Wessels Company). (Quoted on title-page.)

13. ROYAL COMMISSION ON THE HOUSING OF THE WORKING CLASSES. *First Report, P.P. 1884–85*, vol. 30; illustrative extracts may be found in Pike, E. Royston (ed.), *'Busy Times'. Human Documents of the Age of the Forsytes* (New York: Praeger, 1970), pp. 177–92.

14. BOOTH, CHARLES (1902–3). *Life and Labour of the People in London*, 17 vols. (London and New York: Macmillan Co.).

15. ROWNTREE, B. SEEBOHM (n.d.). *Poverty. A Study of Town Life*, 2nd edn (London: Thomas Nelson & Sons).

16. LONDON, JACK (1903). *The People of the Abyss* (London: Macmillan Co.).

17. NEWMAN, GEORGE (1939). *The Building of a Nation's Health* (London: Macmillan Co.), pp. 183–220, 281–359.

18. CRAIG, W. S. (1946). *Child and Adolescent Life in Health and Disease. A Study in Social Paediatrics* (Edinburgh: E. & S. Livingtone Ltd.), pp. 112–205.

19. ROSEN, GEORGE (1958) *A History of Public Health* (New York: MD Publications), pp. 233–49.

20. RIIS, JACOB A. (1892) *The Children of the Poor* (New York: Charles Scribner's Sons).

21. —— (1902) *The Battle with the Slum* (New York: Macmillan Co.).

22. HUNTER, ROBERT (1904). *Poverty* (New York: Macmillan Co.).

23. ROSEN, GEORGE (1953). 'Economic and social policy in the development of public health', *J. Hist. Med.* 7, 406–30.

24. —— (1944). 'The impact of the hospital on the physician, the patient and the community', *Hosp. Admin.* 9, 15–33.

25. PAYNE, GREGORY (1937). *The Control of Tuberculosis in England, Past and Present* (London: Oxford University Press), pp. 9–10.

26. FRAZER, W. M. (1950). *A History of English Public Health, 1834–1939* (London, Bailliere, Tindall and Cox), pp. 71–2.

27. LAMBERT, ROYSTON (1963). *Sir John Simon, 1816–1904, and English Social Administration* (London: MacGilbert and Kee), pp. 250–7, 587–8.

28. DUFFUS, R. L., and HOLT, JR., EMMETT L. (1940). *L. Emmett Holt Pioneer of a Children's Century* (New York: R. Appleton-Century Co.), pp. 175–7.

29. HOFFMAN, F. L. (1921). 'American mortality progress during the last half century', *A Half Century of Public Health*, ed. Ravenel, M. P. (New York: APHA), pp. 95–117.

30. —— (1919). 'Health and national efficiency', *Mod. Med.* 1, 2–3.

31. HILL, H. W. (1919). 'The new public health', ibid. 1, 57–8.

32. DEVINE, EDWARD T. (1910). *Misery and its Causes* (New York: Macmillan Co.), p. 53.

33. *The Health and Sickness of Town Populations . . . District Dispensaries* (1846), pp. 21, 29.

34. *Report of the Commission on the Poor Laws and Relief of Distress*, 3 vols. (London: HMSO, 1909). The Minority Report was issued as vol. 3.

35. WEBB, SIDNEY, and WEBB, BEATRICE (1910). *The State and the Doctor* (London: Longmans Green & Co.).

36. MINISTRY OF HEALTH (1920). Consultative Council on Medical and Allied Services, *Interim Report on the Future Provision of Medical and Allied Services*, Cmd 693 (London).

37. POLITICAL AND ECONOMIC PLANNING (1937). *Report on the British Health Services* (London : PEP).

38. BRITISH HOSPITALS ASSOCIATION (1937). *Report of the Voluntary Hospital Commission* (London : BHA).

39. MINISTRY OF HEALTH (1944). Department of Health for Scotland, *A National Health Service*, Cmd 6502 (London : HMSO), Appendix B.

40. TITMUSS, RICHARD M. (1938). *Poverty and Population. A Factual Study of Contemporary Social Waste* (London, Macmillan Co.).

41. M'GONIGLE, G. C. M., and KIRBY, J. (1936). *Poverty and Public Health* (London : Gollancz).

42. WILKINSON, ELLEN (1939). *The Town that was Murdered. The Life-Story of Jarrow* (London : Victor Gollancz), pp. 236–49.

43. *Our Towns. A Close-Up. A Study made in 1939–1942 with Certain Recommendations by the Hygiene Committee of the Women's Group on Public Welfare . . .* (London : Oxford University Press, 1943).

44. *Hospitals and the State Hospital. Organization and Administration under the National Health Service*, vol. 1, *Background and Blueprint* (London : Acton Society Trust, 1955), p. 14. The reference is to *The Hospital Surveys—The Domesday Book of the Hospital Service* (London : Nuffield Provincial Hospitals Trust, 1946).

45. TITMUSS, RICHARD M. (1950). *Problems of Social Policy* (London : HMSO and Longmans).

46. BEVERIDGE, SIR WILLIAM (1942). *Social Insurance and Allied Services* (American edn) (New York : Macmillan Co.), pp. 158–63.

47. MINISTRY OF HEALTH (1946). *On the State of the Public Health during Six Years of War* (London : HMSO), p. 9.

48. STEVENS, ROSEMARY (1966). *Medical Practice in Modern England* (New Haven : Yale University Press), p. 71.

49. WILSON, N. (1947). *Municipal Health Services* (London : Allen & Unwin).

50. U.S. DEPARTMENT OF HEALTH, EDUCATION, AND WELFARE (1970). *Toward A Social Report*, with an introductory commentary by Cohen, Wilbur J. (University of Michigan), pp. 1–13, 27–40.

51. *Report of the Committee on Local Authority and Allied Personal Social Services*, Cmnd 3703 (London : HMSO, 1970), pp. 120–2 (see particularly p. 120).

52. BERNSTEIN, BETTY J. (1970). 'Public health—Inside or outside the mainstream of the political process? Lessons from the passage of Medicaid', *Am. J. publ. Hlth*, 60, 1690–1700.

53. RANKIN, W. S. (1924). 'Elimination of politics from public health work', *J. Am. med. Ass.* 8, 1285–7.

54. WORLD HEALTH ORGANIZATION (1952). 'Expert Committee on Public Health Administration, First Report', *Technical Report Series*, 55, 5.

55. EVANG, KARL (1960). *Health Service, Society and Medicine* (London : Oxford University Press), pp. 157–8.

56. BROCKINGTON, FRASER (1964). 'A community health service', *Trends in the National Health Service*, ed. Farndale, James (New York, Macmillan Co.), pp. 100–8.

Discussion

With some variation in timing the health services of countries in the Western world have evolved on three distinct lines. First, hospital services originated in religious institutions, but later developed under secular auspices to produce the complex pattern of administration and finance which exists today. Second, medical practice was entirely domiciliary until the eighteenth century, and while its character was profoundly altered by the growth of hospitals, a substantial part of medicine is still practised independently, outside or in association with hospitals. The third strand comprises the public health service, initiated in the second half of the nineteenth century for the control of the physical environment, but later extended to include certain personal health services and, to a limited extent, the treatment of disease. The patchwork of local public health services was not the result of thoughtful planning, but was largely a reflection of the deficiencies of other medical services, both private and public.

The limitations of the traditional pattern of services are everywhere apparent, but are perhaps most conspicuous in countries such as Britain where a national commitment has focused attention on areas of overlap and deficiencies. Obstetric, paediatric, geriatric, and psychiatric services are some which are particularly prejudiced, but there is no part of the health service which is not affected in some degree by the existence of three administrations concerned separately with hospitals, GP services, and public health. With this fragmentation it is impossible to develop a fully comprehensive service which achieves a proper balance between prevention and treatment and between care in and out of hospital.

In Britain the co-ordination of all local health services under a single administration seems inevitable, and has been recommended recently in two Green Papers prepared by the Department of Health and Social Security. While these proposals may be changed in detail and it may be some time before they are implemented, there is little doubt that they indicate the lines on which health services in Britain are likely to develop.

Some points of controversy arising from these proposals, though of particular concern in Britain, are hardly of general interest, for example the responsibilities of the regional health councils and the influence and finance of teaching hospitals under the new administration. Indeed the question whether there should be two or three levels of regional and local administration is one which may have different answers in different countries as may also be the case with finance and organization. There are, however, two issues of wide general interest which in time may confront other countries whose health services are of essentially similar type: (*a*) whether the new authorities should be of an elected or appointed character and (*b*) the training and roles of professional administrators in a unified service.

In Britain it seems clear that the unified health services will be administered by appointed bodies rather than by the elected local authorities. This decision is influenced largely by history, particularly by the fact that GP services developed independently and there would now be strong professional objections to local government control. But in countries where the point of no return has not yet been passed, the question may still be asked whether local health services are best administered by elected bodies.

In favour of this arrangement it is said that it puts the responsibility where it should be, on those who represent the public who pay for the service. On the other side it is objected that the conditions provided by local government are not ideal for health services, an objection illustrated by the failure of the public health service to develop significantly beyond the framework established for it in the nineteenth century. It is possible that under suitable conditions either type of administration might succeed and the pattern may vary from country to country; but perhaps being influenced unduly by their own experience, most doctors in Britain would undoubtedly prefer to accept the advantages and risks associated with an appointed authority.

Inevitably the proposal to unify all health services raises questions concerning the respective roles and training of the public health officer and the hospital administrator. When health services are unified it seems evident that they should be administered by staff trained in all aspects of health services. This requirement is being met for medical staff in Britain by replacement of the traditional public health training leading to the diploma in public health by new courses in health services administration.

What remains unresolved is the more difficult problem of the training and roles of medically qualified and other administrators in the health field. It can hardly be doubted that both are required, the one to deal with problems for which a medical background is desirable and the other with those which require experience in such areas as management and finance. In central government in Britain the respective roles are well defined on lines which apply throughout the Civil Service, and there seems no reason why the same principles should not be incorporated in the district, area, and regional administrations. It would be a valuable step in this direction to make training in health services administration general rather than specialized, and to bring all professional administrators together in a common basic course.

4

EVOLUTION OF MEDICAL PRACTICE

JOHN BROTHERSTON

Evolution of medical practice

Medical care institutions are subject to continuous change in response to pressures of social and scientific events, professional interactions, and state policies. The history of general practice in the United Kingdom illustrates this generalization. One of the many problems in tracing an outline of the story is the changing use of terminology. The different concepts attached to the term general practice at different periods may readily lead to false analogies. The point is not one of simple historical curiosity. There is a risk that a continuing use of the same term may obscure changes so fundamental that they alter the whole basis of the system examined, and place it in danger for lack of examination of its ensuing purpose and requirements. One of the striking features of general practice in more recent times has been the lack of a clear-cut definition of its purpose and requirements. Collings starts out his controversial review of British general practice, made at the beginning of the NHS, by saying:

> General practice is accepted as being something specific, without anyone knowing what it really is. Neither the teacher responsible for instructing future general practitioners nor the specialist who supposedly works in continuous association with the GP, nor for that matter the GP himself, can give an adequate definition of general practice. Though generally identified with the last century concept of 'family doctoring', usually it has ceased to be this. Nevertheless its stability and its reputation rest largely on this identification.
>
> While other branches of medicine have progressed and developed

general practice, instead of developing concurrently, has adapted itself to the changing patterns; and sometimes this adaptation has in fact been regression (1).

In our history general practice emerges as a clear concept in the early nineteenth century. The term was used literally to describe the work of a practitioner who did everything for his patients of which he and medical knowledge were capable, whether medical, surgical, obstetric, or pharmaceutical. The GP was to be a one-man medical service. This simple definition has been subject to steady encroachment by events. Today we use alternative terms such as personal doctor, doctor of first intent, and continuity doctor without very clear definition of our meaning or its consequences. After an earlier period of relative ascendancy, general practice has lost position as a positive concept; it has tended to be the undefined and residual legatee of the medical care estate. Positive definition has tended to be reserved for the things which it shall not do, perhaps without sufficient regard to the coherence, purpose, and requirements of what is left behind.

GENERAL PRACTICE IN THE ASCENDANT

General practice emerged in the early nineteenth century in response to social requirement and developing medical knowledge to meet the needs of a rapidly expanding commercial and industrial community. The story of its emergence is curious and involved. The previously ordained hierarchy of medicine with its tightly defined codes of practice for physicians, surgeons, and apothecaries no longer fitted the needs of the population or the facts of medical knowledge. Holloway has summarized this system (2):

'The law', wrote J. E. Willcock in 1830, 'recognizes only three orders of the medical profession: physicians, surgeons, and apothecaries.' Between the physician, who could claim to belong to a learned profession, the surgeon, who practised a craft, and the apothecary, who followed a trade, the gap was wide and impassable. Chief Justice Best pointed out, in 1828, that 'the distinction between the various departments of the medical art' had been drawn 'with great precision'. Each practitioner 'is protected in his own branch, and neither must interfere with the province of the other'. This system of stratification was not only ancient, it was also peculiarly rigid. In the eighteenth century, no apothecary could secure the licence of the Surgeons' Company unless he first withdrew his membership of the Society of Apothecaries. Even as late as 1834 it was necessary for members of the College of Surgeons and licentiates of the Society of Apothecaries to be disfranchised before qualifying as licentiates of the College of Physicians. The medical profession, it was held, had its ranks and orders, each with their own function and sphere of usefulness; and each estate had its necessary position of subordination and authority. Bishop Butler's view that the Architect of the Universe had 'distributed men into different ranks, and at the same time united them into one society' was applicable to the medical profession as to society in general.

Later Rivington referred to this as 'the age of small, but not entirely independent sovereignties—the age of the Medical Heptarchy. This primitive condition was not changed for more than 300 years' (3). In fact the process of change had already begun long before the declared emergence of the GP in the nineteenth century. The apothecary was providing general medical attention for the rapidly growing population of London, and surgeons were extending their practice by prescription of drugs long before this. The term general practice was first coined in the early eighteenth century, although it did not come into common use till more than a century later (4–6). By 1830 a correspondent in the *London Medical Gazette* was to state: 'We are a body of men who exist because the wants of society have raised us up. The pure practitioners of surgery, or of obstetrics, can subsist only in a populous city . . . there is room for one physician only, where there may be twenty general practitioners' (2).

The changes which occurred in the structure of the medical profession after 1800 were summed up in the preface to the 1847 *London and Provincial Medical Directory*. Describing the gradations of the medical profession it states (2):

The Physician, the Surgeon, and the Apothecary mark its subdivisions; and law and custom would seem distinctly to have defined the position and duties of each class. It is needless to observe, however, that practically this classification has become almost obsolete. The nomenclature alone remains in force, and its inapplicability to the existing state of things constitutes an admirable *argumentum ad absurdum* for the reorganization of the profession. In times past, these several practitioners, in their various grades, were no doubt equal to the sanatory requirements of the people . . . At all events, in the present age, the public, advanced in knowledge and power, perceive that they are considerably benefited by a departure from the economy of the profession as ordered of old. A change, accordingly, is now in progress, which, like all transitions, is marked by a confusion of position and character among individual members, that calls for some state interference to establish order and union in a profession which has thus been disturbed, and to meet the increasing demands for excellence by a people rapidly progressing themselves. If we look around, indeed, it will be found that the Physician, the Surgeon, and the Apothecary, as distinct and separate practitioners, exist but little more than their several designations . . . For whilst Physicians, and Surgeons, and Apothecaries, appear to be so vitally interested in the continuance of useless titles, they really are, by the force of a public convenience they cannot withstand, being gradually classed into Consulting and General Practitioners . . .

The emergence of the GP across the tightly ordained lines of earlier arrangements illustrates the pressures of social need and technical change on traditional organizations. Later similar processes to those which brought the GP into being were to operate to circumscribe his own role and functions. There is another feature of these developments with considerable interest for us today. The nineteenth-century GP emerged from a variety of backgrounds, which gave general practice from the start a range of characteristics of quality, scope, and regional variation which in some senses persist up to the present time. It is almost as if there were some process of professional inheritance from one practitioner to his successor combined with persistence of tradition and social pressures which facilitates the survival of high standards in some situations and low standards in others. In its origins, despite the common concept that the GP was to practise all aspects of medicine, the diversity of origins gave rise to a range of performance which already promised to obscure a clear definition of the nature and purposes of general practice in the future.

The earlier emergence of the apothecary as a prototype general practitioner was given statutory force by the Apothecaries Act of 1815 which enabled the Worshipful Company to give form and substance to an appropriate education for the emerging practitioners. Coinciding with the general movement of reform and change in professional institutions to meet the needs of a prospering industrial society, and the desires of an enlarging middle class for appropriate careers for their sons, it helped to promote the emergence of a new class of better-educated practitioners, who later would be active in the movement for medical reform (7–8).

Paradoxically the stereotyping of the GP as an apothecary had opposite effects in so far as it associated the GP with what was the lowest order in the medical hierarchy. The debates on medical reform and unification of the medical profession were long tinged with arguments about the necessity to preserve an inferior order of practitioner to meet the needs of the poorer classes. The view of general practice as the lowest order in the medical world persisted long after the statutory decision to unify the profession.

The surgeon was another noteworthy ancestor of the GP. It became common practice for the embryo practitioner in England to seek both membership of the College of Surgeons and the licence of apothecary. Wakley ceaselessly propagated the view in the *Lancet* that the future lay with the surgeons of England. There were many GPs who preferred to call themselves surgeons (9). The common use of the term surgery to describe the doctors' consulting rooms to this day is a reminder that many GPs then and for long afterwards saw themselves as surgeons, and their professional self-esteem and skill lay in that field of practice. This too had its significance for the future.

Another source of GPs was the Scottish universities. In the earlier part of the nineteenth century Edinburgh University had perhaps the most ambitious requirements for medical education. In 1825 the curriculum was extended from three to four years (10). About half of the graduates came from England, returning there with their MD. Many of them established themselves as provincial physicians like Charles Hastings, the founding father of the British Medical Association. Few of the provincial physicians could practise as 'pures', i.e. solely as consultants. No doubt few of them dispensed drugs, the hallmark of the apothecary GP. But most of them were GPs in effect. All the Edinburgh graduates studied surgery and midwifery as well as medicine for their degree. In Scotland itself the majority of GPs were university graduates. The Royal Commission on the Medical Acts which reported in 1882 was told that the proportion at that date was two-thirds.

The emerging GPs were diverse in their education, their social organizations, and no doubt in the nature and quality of their work. Some would be indistinguishable from the élite physicians and surgeons, and might still spurn the title of GP, although in fact doing general practice. Some at the lower end of the apothecary spectrum might be as much shopkeeprs as practitioners. Later in 1879 Rivington classified GPs into a number of orders which merged into each other (11):

I—The dispensing order, which is distinguished by the fact of supplying medicines to patients, may be again subdivided into two chief groups or sub-orders—(*a*) The surgeon-chemist, or the red-bottle and blue-bottle practitioners, who combine the work of medical men with the retail business of a chemist. An open shop is kept with glass-cases containing toothbrushs, nailbrushes, patent medicines, seidlitz powders, Eno's fruit salt, soap, scents, delectable lozenges, chest protecters and feeding bottles. The retail trade is the great source of emolument, and could not be given up without serious damage to the business. (*b*) The surgeon-apothecary, with an open surgery and a red lamp. No retail trade is done, but advice and a bottle of physic is given for a moderate sum—a shilling is a common charge in the poorer neighbourhoods. A few in this and the preceding group keep medical dispensaries, and attend patients for a small weekly payment varying from 2d to 1s. As the scale is ascended the surgery retires more and more into the background, until it reaches the interior of the dwelling, where it is no longer exposed to the vulgar gaze. At last it disappears entirely, and the second sub-order is attained, or—
II—The non-dispensing or consultant order. Medicine is prescribed, the prescriptions being made up at a chemist's. Patients are seen and visited at a lower fee than that of the regular physician. Half a guinea is often charged. Members of the non-dispensing order are found at

fashionable watering places. They shade off on the one hand into the highest of the dispensing order, and on the other into the regular consulting physician.

The range of quality of Victorian general practice must have been enormous. Mapother in one of the Carmichael essays supplies the following quotation from Carmichael (12):

> The following placard is copied, verbatim, from a board which the author saw suspended, during the summer of 1839, at the window of an apothecary's shop in Manchester. Such notifications exhibit so extraordinary a melange as to excite the astonishment and ridicule of foreigners but are so common in Great Britain that their incongruity passes unheeded by all classes of Englishmen: 'A B Surgeon and Apothecary. Prescriptions and family medicines accurately compounded. Teeth extracted at one shilling each. Women attended in labour 2s 6d each. Patent medicines and perfumery. Best London pickles. Fish sauces. Bear's grease. Soda water. Ginger beer. Lemonade. Congreve matches, and Warren's blackening.' I inquired of the proprietor of this heterogeneous mass if he really was, as his placard announced, a surgeon and apothecary? He candidly acknowledged that he had no right to call himself a surgeon, but stated that he was a licentiate of the Apothecaries' Company of London, and therefore legally qualified to practise medicine.

The example is perhaps grotesque, but it illustrates one end of the tradition. There were also the practitioners of mass medicine; the sixpenny and shilling doctors who attempted to assuage the endless thirst of the British people for medicines with strong-tasting, highly coloured waters. There were the club and Poor Law practitioners who struggled to care for their flock in circumstances of extreme difficulty if not degradation.

Bernard Shaw's caricatures of the GP in the preface to *The Doctor's Dilemma* had a basis in fact.

> To make matters worse doctors are hideously poor . . . Better be a railway porter than an ordinary English general practitioner.

> To secure the vehement and practically unanimous support of the rank and file of the medical profession for any sort of treatment or operation, all that is necessary is that it can be easily practised by a rather shabbily dressed man in a surgically dirty house without any assistance and that the materials for it shall cost say, a penny (13).

There are also many examples at the other end of the scale. McConaghey has given an interesting picture of practice during the times of James MacKenzie. Sir James MacKenzie was not outwardly an exceptional recruit to general practice. In 1878 it was certainly not uncommon for a Scottish graduate who had won two gold medals at his university to believe there was no option for him but general practice. Nor do I suppose that the partnership he entered in Burnley was exceptional. The senior partner, Henry Briggs, had been a demonstrator in anatomy in University College Hospital and graduated MD of London before going to Burnley in 1855. The other partner, John Brown, was a cousin of the author of *Rab and His Friends*. He had studied medicine in Aberdeen graduating MD with honours and ChM with highest honours in 1863. Subsequently he had practised for ten years in South Africa before returning to Edinburgh to become Lister's dresser and a demonstrator in anatomy at the University. In 1877 he took the diploma of public health of Cambridge and in 1878 the FRCS of England. About the practice James MacKenzie wrote: '... Our practice comprised all classes, the bulk being of the working class. It was an old-fashioned practice of many years standing, and we followed the old custom of dispensing our own medicines. It will be seen that the type of practice was not of a very elevated order ...' The practice was certainly general in the original sense of the term. MacKenzie had regular surgical duties as well as obstetric and medical practice. In discussing pain later he wrote:

> In operating on ovarian cysts for instance, if I found that the abdominal wall was not tender, nor the muscle rigid, then I knew I would meet with no troublesome adhesions. If, however, the abdominal wall was hard and tender, I would certainly meet with adhesions. But these observations were too few to enable me to speak with assurance on this point.

We should also note that MacKenzie was one of the founding members of the staff of the Burnley Hospital which was opened in 1886 (14).

Sir Heneage Ogilvie was not describing a myth when in looking back to the end of the nineteenth century he wrote in 1953:

There was no essential separation between the doctor who looked after the patient at home and the doctor who looked after him in hospital . . . Practitioners were seeing the same cases, using the same methods of investigation, giving the same treatment, doing the same operations, and using the same language as members of the hospital staff (15).

1858 AND UNIFICATION OF THE MEDICAL PROFESSION

In addition to the protracted and involved debates on medical reform the period 1830–58 had seen great change and improvement in basic standards of medical education, and the quality of individuals emerging as GPs. Charles Newman claims that the groundwork for reform of medical education had been effectively laid before the establishment of the General Medical Council by the Medical Act in 1858 (10). The point is striking if uncharitable towards the later work of the Council; and it is common enough that reforms take place only when the parties concerned are already well on the way to the objective. More will be said about medical education later, but probably to contemporaries the outstanding achievement of the Act of 1858 was the official unification of all the medical castes and septs into one profession of registered medical practitioners. In an official memorandum written in 1858, in explanation of the Bill, John Simon then medical officer of the General Board of Health had stated that there were five main objects which members of the medical profession desire to be realized by any legislation (16):

1. 'Qualified medical practitioners' should be legally defined, and only such practitioners should be competent to hold any public medical appointments, to give any medical certificates, or to cover fees for medical attendance.

2. That an authentic Register be kept for annual publication of all legally qualified medical practitioners.

3. That it be made an offence for any person 'falsely to assume a title or description' implying him to be a legally qualified medical practitioner.

4. That the names of persons 'guilty of certain disgraceful offences' be removable from the Register.

5. That the legally qualified medical practitioner be entitled to practise equally in all parts of the United Kingdom without hindrance from any local restrictions.

Rivington, looking back from 1879 with a critical eye at the outcome of the Medical Act of 1858, had no doubt of the benefits achieved in removing the anomalies which separated the professsion (12):

Before the Medical Act of 1858 was passed by Parliament the grossest anomalies prevailed throughout the United Kingdom in the relative position of the Licensing Bodies to each other, and in the privileges of the various orders of Medical Practitioners. England, Ireland, and Scotland had different interests. The colleges waged war against the Universities, and at the same time were at variance both with the Apothecaries Societies and with each other. Exclusive privileges were possessed by the Medical Corporations, and special local jurisdictions in cities and provinces were assigned to them which none could invade without being exposed to a rigorous prosecution.

The emergence of the numerous and vigorous class of GPs had provided the strength of the medical reform movement. They saw no reason for the restrictive practices, and the territorial limitations of the old order were in any case contrary to the prevailing *laissez-faire* political philosophy. The desire for some expression of corporate professional life had banded together provincial practitioners in the Provincial and Medical Surgical Association which was founded by Charles Hastings in Worcester in 1832 and which became the British Medical Association in 1855. In the end the sober and steady statesmanship of the Association took a leading role in asking for a single registering authority and a uniform medical qualification, 'entitling the holder to practise in any part of the Kingdom, and in any branch of the profession' (8).

The Association was meeting in Edinburgh when the Act became law and at a celebration dinner Sir Charles Hastings said (17):

Forty years ago, and after having passed through the different examinations required by the University of Edinburgh, I crossed the Tweed; but no sooner had I passed over the border, than I lost all the advantage of having gone through my full curriculum of study here, and passing through all my examinations. In fact, I became an illegal practitioner and I have remained so right up to this present hour (laughter and cheers).

Today we may take for granted the concept of a unified profession with one standard of basic education and registration, but prior to the Act argument had been raised in favour of a lower order of practitioner more plentiful and cheaply produced to meet the needs of the poor and rural populations. The British Medical Association had earnestly countered such arguments in its memorandum of evidence (17):

> Every attempt to create an inferior grade of medical men of limited education and with aptitude only for the 'ordinary exigencies' of practice should be resisted. Disease affected people wherever they were and of whatever class they were, and so the same degree of medical skill should be available for everyone.

So ended a movement to introduce a *feldscher* level of practitioner in the United Kingdom. The acceptance of a united profession with one standard of entry to license was to have profound and continuing effects on medical education and its relationship to general practice.

SPECIALIZATION: THE RISE AND FALL OF THE GENERAL PRACTITIONER SPECIALIST

> Whereas the theme of medical history in the nineteenth century was the integration of diverse skills into one medical profession, the theme of the twentieth century medical practice has been a fragmentation within the profession (18).

The later years of the nineteenth century foreshadow subsequent developments of specialized practice in medicine and surgery. Rivington in his 1888 Carmichael Essay on the Medical Profession described the scene at that time (3):

> Small portions of physic and surgery have been separated from the parent trunks, and been consigned to groups of practitioners, who are hence known as specialists. The eye engages the entire attention of oculists or ophthalmic surgeons; the ear of aurists or aural surgeons; the mind of lunacy doctors or practitioners, or alienists;

deformities fall to the orthopaedic surgeons . . . Another distinct branch has been made out of diseases of the skin, and the practitioners in skin diseases are known as skin doctors, or dermatologists. The larynx, or part of 'the throat', was only a few years ago severed from the rest of the body, and its diseases were made into a speciality, owing to the necessity for using a new instrument, styled the laryngoscope, for their recognition and treatment. This was literally 'holding up the mirror to nature' . . . Some surgeons give their entire attention to diseases of the urinary organs, especially to stone stricture, etc.; others to venereal complaints . . . Many physicians and surgeons 'take up' as it is termed some favourite subjects, or the diseases of some particular organ other than those already mentioned; thus there is the specialist in diseases of the nervous system, or the neurologist, the fever specialist, the specialist in gout and rheumatism, the specialist in cancer, the specialist for the heart, the specialist for the lungs, the specialist for idiocy, the specialist for the liver, the specialist for the stomach, the specialist for ovariotomy, the operating surgeon or specialist, the specialist for cleft palate, the specialist for the rectum, the specialist for the male generative organs, the specialist for the kidneys, and the specialist for children's diseases.

These were early signs of change. It was not till later that multiplication of specialties seriously impinged on general practice. The great acceleration of specialization was a product mainly of twentieth-century science and technology. Emphasis shifts from the generalist to the generalist with a special interest, and from him in turn to the full-time specialist. Specialization by concentrating effort and skill and by enlarging experience in a narrow field brought great gains in knowledge and patient care. It also created problems of organization and communication within the profession (18).

The GP mirrored the response of the profession as a whole. Already to a small extent before the First World War, and particularly between the wars, some GPs were adding to their general practice specialist work in some limited field, and a variety of diplomas were available to give direction to their learning and testimony to their skill. It was natural that this should happen. In many parts of this country there was no one else to do the work. There was no outside definition of a specialist. So there came into existence the GP ophthalmologist, anaesthetist, ENT specialist, radiologist, and so on. Possibilities of development were limited by time and hospital facilities. The possibilities were also financially circumscribed because NHI which had changed the scene radically so far as payment of basic practice was concerned, made only marginal provision for payment of special skills (18).

This era of the GP specialist was ended by the NHS, which replaced him with a service of consultant specialists deployed throughout the country. The interest of noting this earlier reflex response of general practice to new pressures, is not to regret the past. The development of widely available consultant specialist services has been perhaps the greatest single achievement of the NHS. It is to record an outlet which existed previously for the aspirations and skills of the GP. This outlet has been closed perhaps without sufficient regard to the consequences.

THE GENERAL PRACTITIONER SURGEON

Much the largest field of work for the GP which we would now call specialist was in surgery. It has already been noted that the surgeon was one of the main stems from which the GP originated. Many GPs had thought of themselves as surgeons and called themselves surgeons. Until the passing of the Medical Act in 1858 the College of Surgeons probably had more influence in the profession than any other single medical body in England and Wales (7). Previous to the Act there had been an influential body of GPs who wished to see GPs wholly enfranchised within the College of Surgeons (7). In 1886 in England out of a total of 25,998 on the medical register, 17,876 were recorded as Members of the College of Surgeons and 1,124 were Fellows (3). Before and for long after the passing of the Act medical education whose objective was to produce the safe GP, was a good deal concerned with surgery, including surgical anatomy and operative technique.

Macnamara has given a picture of earlier teaching and practice based on lecture notes taken in Dublin in 1838–42 and 1856–8 (19). Before anaesthetic or antisepsis the body cavities were sacrosanct except for paracetesis.

Surgery consisted of dealing with fractures, dislocations, and other injuries, and as best one could with strangulated hernia, hydrocele, aneurisms of the vessels in the limbs, knowing how to pass a catheter and possibly being able to trephine. Owing to the rather ebullient temperament of our fellow countrymen, the faction fights and the classical misuse of the shillelagh at country fairs, there can have been no shortage of depressed fractures of the skull to be treated, and the trephine must have been much in use. I think it is not too imaginative to state that some at least of our fellow practitioners were pretty skilled in its use. Surely they did not lack for practice.

Prostatic enlargement was presumably just as common as it is today and gonorrheal stricture vastly commoner, so the catheter must have been in great demand, and skill in its use of great value to the practitioner. Much sound advice is given in the notes as to its use, and great stress laid on the importance of avoiding false passages. They also emphasize the wisdom of having a finger in the rectum to guide it on its way.

A doctor uncle of mine told me that when he was a boy, he well remembered the scene in the kitchen of his home in Corofin on the evening of a fair day. It would be full of elderly men sitting around on chairs, in various stages of discomfort waiting for his father to come along and catheterize them. When this was successfully accomplished they would depart to their respective homes. There was, of course, no alternative to catheter life in those days.

GP surgery was a significant activity up until the arrival of the National Health Service in 1948. Bradford Hill recorded that in 1938–9, 2·5 million surgical operations were performed by GPs, an average of three per doctor per week (18).

The importance that surgery had had for many GPs was noted by Collings (1). He describes his visit to a cottage hospital where GP surgery still survived in the first months of the NHS. Although it was a Saturday afternoon about half the doctors in the area were there, 'They were looking at X-ray films, discussing cases, and exhibiting an enthusiasm which was really remarkable.' Nine of the ten beds were surgical. All the interest was in difficult surgical cases. In contrast a severely ill medical patient was not discussed.

One of the great advances of the NHS has been the virtual replacement of independent GP surgery by the specialist surgeon. No one would wish to change that picture. But Collings notes (1) that when he discussed the place of the GP with hospital authorities, 'They drew attention to the crimes of the G.P. working in a cottage hospital. Most of them expressed their determination to eliminate the G.P. surgeon. This seemed to be their focal point in thinking about general practice.'

We can only note that the passing of independent GP surgery must have been a major blow to the assumptions and self-esteem of an important sector of general practice. Abruptly for better or worse on that account alone general practice ceased to be general in the original sense. Essential administration amputations administered for the best possible reasons may have debilitating side-effects.

THE GENERAL PRACTITIONER AND THE HOSPITAL

In the earlier days of general practice the hospital was not significant for the great bulk of medical care however severe the circumstances. Indeed until this century hospitals probably increased rather than diminished risk in severe illness or surgical treatment. It was in that sense of little importance whether or not a GP had access to hospital beds. He could deliver his obstetric cases more safely at home, and operate more safely on the kitchen table.

During the whole of the period reviewed the teaching hospitals were under control of consultant physicians, surgeons, and obstetricians. The growing number of large voluntary hospitals in larger towns tended to follow the same pattern, although well into this century some of them were staffed by men who also engaged in general practice. GPs worked on a part-time salaried basis in Poor Law and other municipal institutions, but meagre remuneration and poor working facilities tended to make this a bitter chore in the professional memory rather than any kind of privilege. Three phases of relationship between the GP and the hospital call for special comment.

a. 'Hospital abuse'

From the early days of general practice as the recognized source of medical care for the large majority of the population, there was the making of a conflict with hospital colleagues in the large centres where out-patient services were developed. The issue was intensified with the creation of special hospitals, whose out-patient departments it was alleged, were used by middle-class patients who could well afford to pay a GP. The various Carmichael Prize essays on the medical profession written in the last quarter of the nineteenth century return to the point that hospital out-patient departments are under-cutting the GP and doing him out of his rightful and very necessary earnings. For example Hardy reported (20):

During the last few years enquiries have been made among a number of general practitioners practising in and around London as to the effect which the hospital out-patient system has on their practices, and from the replies received it appears that there is general agreement that it is very prejudicial—(1) by treating patients who can afford to pay the small fees asked for in many of the districts, or who could join provident dispensaries; (2) by the absence of adequate enquiry into the social circumstances of patients; (3) by the treatment of trivial complaints; and (4) by depriving the general practitioner of those cases, the treatment of which would be of service to him in maintaining his professional efficiency. One general practitioner in the East End of London writes that out-patient departments compete with the general practitioner by taking from him his bread and butter, treating gratuitously those well able to pay for medical attendance at home. Another from South London writes that a large number of working people in that part of London pay for medical attendance at the rate of one shilling for medicine at the doctor's surgery, and one shilling and sixpence for a visit and medicine. If they can get free advice and medicine at a hospital of course they will go there, but he finds that they will not put themselves out to go. In bad weather they send for the general practitioner, or go to him for medicine. In fine weather they all flock to the hospitals. Another from the S.W. district writes that minor surgery is almost unknown in his practice beyond opening an abcess, extracting a needle, or stitching up a cut, and even these small operations are very rare. Circumcisions and removal of tonsils all go to hospitals. Where a fee of a shilling is charged, he says, as at some hospitals, it is in direct competition with the general practitioner. One shilling, he adds, is his own most frequent fee for consultation and medicine. When it is remembered that one million and a half of persons are reported to be treated at the London Hospitals, general and special, it will be seen what difficulties general practitioners who are even willing to accept such low fees as 1s 6d for visit and medicine, have to contend with in earning a living, for it is quite incredible that in the richest city in the world one out of three of its inhabitants should be unable to pay such modest fees as these.

Rosemary Stevens notes that complaints of such 'hospital abuse' recur in the *British Medical Journal* from the 1850s. The issue was crucial to the development of medical practice. A possible solution suggested by the British Medical Association was open access by all practitioners to hospital beds. If this had happened our system of practice might have been the same as in the United States. Instead the 'referral' system was developed. From this acrimonious dispute developed our unique convention that the specialist must only see patients referred by a GP. It developed from informal professional agreement; it has become the main-spring of our medical care system. In Stevens's words 'The physician and surgeon retained the hospital, but the general practitioner retained the patient' (18). Later as the importance of the hospital in the medical care system steadily enlarged, questions were to be asked whether the GP really can retain the patient without some stake in the hospital.

b. The cottage hospital

It has been noted that GPs were gradually displaced from the larger voluntary hospitals, even outside the teaching centres. The separation of much urban general practice from the hospital dates from long before the NHS. In smaller towns cottage hospitals developed. The first was created in the 1850s. These grew in number up until the outbreak of the Second World War. They were essentially GP hospitals, where practitioners in suburban, small town, and rural practice could admit their patients. Their development in this century was in some ways analagous to the development of the GP specialist. He attempted to provide a parallel service to the consultant specialist. As the hospital became more essential to patient care, a complete service of general practice required its own hospitals. That they were a stimulus and an asset to the GP is not in doubt. Collings, in his general criticism of British general practice in other circumstances, notes with approval the quality of practice where the practitioners were linked to cottage hospitals. The reputation and future of the cottage hospital was, however, clouded by some of the GP surgery practised there. Hence Ogilvie when making his eloquent plea for GP beds in the NHS discussed some special circumstances of abuse in the past, which had led to a misplaced condemnation of cottage hospitals in principle (15):

> As a direct result of the complete separation of the general practitioner from the hospital, there had developed in many cottage hospitals and in some voluntary hospitals in the smaller towns a policy of excluding all but general practitioners. Such a policy which was quite frankly mercenary, and had for its main object the retention among a local group of the emoluments and benefits of the private beds, was to a large extent responsible for the artificial and, as it turned out, disastrous barrier erected by the National Health Service Act between the practitioners and the hospitals. I will cite the imaginary town of X, situated in lovely country at a distance of thirty miles from the manufacturing city and university town of Y. With the development of motor transport X had become a dormitory, where all the wealthy men who earn their money in Y had their country houses. The X War Memorial Hospital was their particular pride. Its buildings were the latest thing in hospital architecture; its equipment was the best that money could buy. Two of the hospital rules were significant. First, that no one might be elected to the hospital staff till he had been in practice in the neighbourhood for a minimum of five years; and, second, that no patient might be treated except by a member of the staff. The first rule excluded anyone with higher degrees, or at any rate with adequate postgraduate training, from appointment to the staff; in practice it meant that staff appointments were for sale, since the purchase of a partnership often included a guarantee of such an appointment. The second rule denied to patients treatment by experts of their own choice—indeed, treatment by experts at all if an expert be defined as one who has made a whole-time study of the art that he practises.
>
> The standard of work in hospitals of the type I have mentioned was in some instances quite deplorable, particularly where surgery was concerned. In the view of many at the time the Act was under discussion, the occurrence of disasters amply justified the closing of cottage hospitals. How wrong this opinion was we have since learned to our cost.

Hospital surveys carried out during the Second World War were influential in shaping hospital policy under the NHS. In one of these it was noted (21):

> The high proportion of surgical cases dealt with at the small 'general practitioner' hospitals is very striking. Largely no doubt it is a reflection of the general shortage of hospital beds for the acute sick, the effect being that the surgical case, which is often urgent and must be admitted, crowds out the medical case which should properly be admitted for diagnosis and observation or treatment but is not so urgent. Other factors may be responsible in some hospitals, such as the presence in the district of one or more practitioners with a flair for surgery, or the preference of the nursing staff for the more interesting surgical case. Whatever the reason may be, the result is unfortunate, since in some instances it involves surgery by general practitioners whose skill and experience must necessarily be limited, and since in all instances it represents a diversion of this type of hospital from its proper function, namely the nursing under the care of their own general practitioner of medical and minor surgical cases which cannot properly be nursed at home.

c. The hospital before and after the National Health Service

Any impressions that all or most GPs possessed hospital privileges before 1948 or that none do today would be equally wrong. The exact picture is not clear but probably about one in five GPs had hospital beds in the late 1930s, with or without a speciality interest, mostly in cottage or small hospitals. Although the proportion of practitioners with direct control of beds in cottage hospitals is now only about one in ten, another one in five have attachments with hospitals as part-time clinical assistants to consultants or some similar capacity (18). The proportion of GPs with some hospital connection may therefore be slightly greater than before the NHS. It is probable, however, that the contact is less intense, and also the range of responsibility. Another change should also be observed. Before 1948 the GP could move his place of work by purchase of another practice. The successful practitioner in an industrial area without hospital privileges could move to a suburb or county town where he would have access to hospital beds. There was an informal incentive in the system. Some moved, some never got beyond the aspiration, but even that had perhaps some value (22).

In some ways the issue today is more important than in the past. The hospital has become increasingly important as the centre of stimulus and professional interaction in the medical care system. In addition surveys of hospital patients have raised the question whether a variously estimated proportion of patients in NHS specialist hospital beds really require specialist care; or whether they might not equally well or better be looked after by their own practitioner in simpler surroundings. There has been a continuously recurring debate since the earliest days of the NHS whether we do not pay too high a price for the tidiness of our system of closed hospital staffing with consultant specialists: a price impossible to reckon except by conjecture, but paid in terms of professional separation of consultant and GP, loss of stimulus to the GP, and loss of knowledge of the outside world to the specialist.

Collings in his survey of practice recorded a bleak picture of separation between hospital and practitioner: 'I find it hard to imagine any circumstances which would more effectively isolate the general practitioner from the specialists and the hospital services than the circumstances now prevailing in most of the areas I visited' (1).

Shortly afterwards another survey of general practice was made by Hadfield who reported in 1953 in much less critical and abrasive terms, but he too noted separation and isolation of the parts of the service (23):

> My foremost impression is that lack of unity in the NHS and lack of unity in the medical profession. Both of these are jeopardizing the status and the effectiveness of general practice. I became aware, early on, that unless certain gaps are closed the patient will not derive maximum benefit from the Service. The human gaps must be closed. The general practitioner, the consultant, and the public health medical officer need to get to know each other and then to learn to work in concert. There is growing up a new generation of consultants and a still newer one of those who will become consultants. These know little of the general practitioner and are unaware of his difficulties. Neither are they aware how easily these difficulties may be increased. Then the public health service and the

general practitioner service seem to be treading different paths. Where their paths meet there is often doubt and misunderstanding.

Since that time efforts have been made to close the gap, for example by the establishment of clinical assistantships in hospital, by the development of direct access to hospital diagnostic facilities, and by the creation of local hospital-based postgraduate educational activities.

Sir Heneage Ogilvie in a paper already noted, discussing the historical separation of the GP from the hospital, said (15):

> At the present time much of the educative value of practice is lost to the practitioner because he is unable to pursue his investigations to the point where a firm diagnosis is possible, or to treat his patients when they require nursing. On the other hand, the hospitals are inundated with cases of a comparatively trivial nature that the practitioner should have treated, and in examinations that he could just as well have made himself. The answer lies in the provision of general practitioner beds.

In the same number of the *British Medical Journal*, J. G. M. Hamilton commented (24):

> A most significant result of these hospital developments has been to withdraw from the GP many of his patients at the times of greatest clinical interest and to deny him the professional satisfaction of a good therapeutic job done. I hold that nothing has done more than this to promote the much discussed decline in the status of the GP and to turn him into a purveyor of certificates, a finger-post to hospital, and a prescriber of minor ailments.

John Hunt, the founder of the Royal College of General Practioners, stated his views in 1961. He drew attention to seven major reports of government or professional committees which had each in varying terms recommended that the GP must be drawn more closely into hospital work. He acknowledged the good intentions and some efforts made but asked if much more could not be done. Specifically he stated that the simplest and most effective link would be the creation of GP beds, where practitioners could look after their own patients. He asked, can GPs take full responsibility for some of their patients in hospital? And answered (25):

Medical schools teach students to treat patients in hospital. All doctors entering general practice in Great Britain now must have spent a year in preregistration hospital appointments or have been registrars or senior hospital medical officers, and have gained post-graduate degrees and diplomas. Ther are now more than enough family doctors with the D.Obst.R.C.O.G. for the number of general-practitioner maternity beds. One-fifth of those now entering general practice have held a registrar's appointment, and it seems wasteful that their training and experience in hospital work should not be of continuing benefit to their own patients later. Family doctors already undertake full responsibility for treating their patients at home, and there can be no doubt that many of them are capable of taking equal responsibility for some of these same patients during short spells in hospital.

In retrospect the most significant development in the history of British general practice arose from the professional consensus arrived at around the beginning of this century that the demarcation of responsibility between the urban GP and consultant was to take place at the gates of the city hospital. The convention was formed at a time when the hospital was not yet essential to medical care. Perhaps it was for this reason that such a convention could be reached. Subsequent events which shaped general practice such as the introduction of NHI were directed on this assumption, and underpinned it by methods of remuneration which rewarded the practitioner for patient care only in his consulting room or the patient's home, and which gave no incentive to carry his skills into hospital.

Two consequences followed. Home-based general practice was preserved. We were insulated from subsequent pressures towards universal specialization which have eroded the cadre of GPs in other countries. To be sweeping, it is to this that we owe the asset of a numerically strong front line service of practitioners.

On the other hand as the hospital increased in importance the practitioner was shut out from an institution essential for complete patient care. General practice in the original sense would no longer be possible for the urban practitioner. More significant in the long run was the loss of potential professional stimulus through sharing the scientific environment of the hospital, and a risk of increasing separation of specialist and general care.

PUBLIC POLICY AND GENERAL PRACTICE

We have seen how pressures of medical development and associated changes in professional work eroded the original specification of general practice. Similar processes to those which had brought forth the all-purpose doctor gradually operated against him. In parallel with these trends public policy had an important influence in supporting the run of events. The first major event of public policy affecting general practice was the introduction of NHI after 1911; this provided a practitioner for all insured wage-earners. It contributed little positive to the definition of general practice. Its negative effects on the development of specialist work by the practitioner have already been noted. On the other hand events after 1911 enormously influenced the direction and social circumstances of practice. Although NHI came to be widely accepted by public and profession alike, there was also a running fire of criticism throughout its existence. This was not entirely captious or self-interested; some of the best practitioners were most critical of its alleged failure to reward quality. Its main effect on the profession was to raise the level of work at the lower end of practice and to give a greatly increased measure of financial security to the doctor. Later Sir George Newman discussed the report of the Royal Commission set up in 1924 to examine the workings of NHI (26):

> It is instructive to observe that the evidence given to the Commission by the British Medical Association included the following words:
>
> (*a*) Large numbers, indeed whole classes of persons are now receiving a real medical attention which they formerly did not receive at all.
>
> (*b*) The number of practitioners in proportion to the population in densely populated areas has increased.

(*c*) The amount and character of the medical attention given is superior to that formerly given in the best of the old clubs, and immensely superior to that given in the great majority of the clubs which were far from the best.

(*d*) Illness is now coming under skilled observation and treatment at an earlier stage than was formerly the case.

(*e*) Speaking generally, the work of the practitioners has been given a bias towards prevention, which was formerly not so marked.

(*f*) Clinical records have been, or are being, provided which may be made of great service in relation to medical research and public health.

(*g*) Co-operation among practitioners is being encouraged to an increasing degree.

(*h*) There is now a more marked recognition than formerly of the collective responsibility of the profession to the community in respect of all health matters.

Much the most remarkable analysis of medical care needs for the future in the post First World War era was contained in the report of the Dawson Committee set up in 1920 by the Ministry of Health (27). Here indeed was an attempt to define the purpose and needs of a comprehensive medical care system, and its component and interlinked front and second lines. The GP should be provided with a primary health centre, which was foreseen as a GP hospital and diagnostic centre, to be provided amongst other facilities with radiology, laboratory, and a common-room to serve as a meeting-place for GPs of the district. Here he would work with other practitioners and specialist colleagues.

No small part of the advantage likely to follow from such institutional provision would be the raising of the standard of professional efficiency. Medical knowledge has far outstripped the means for its application. Within the hospital the student studies the problems of disease under favourable circumstances; he has near at hand, not only the equipment of the ward, but the laboratories of radiography, pathology, and chemistry; he can marshal his observations, and follow up results. Under existing conditions he leaves hospital for practice, and there is a sudden drop to the limited opportunities attached to the crowded surgery and the patient's home, and the more medical knowledge advances the bigger the drop becomes. In the Health Centre there would be the equipment and the encouragement to do good work, and opportunities for observation and investigation and self-improvement. Disease, too, would be detected in its earlier and, therefore, more curable stages. Judged alone by the effect on medical men and medical knowledge, it would be impossible to exaggerate the benefits that would accrue to the community by the establishment of these Health Centres.

The report lies on the table as a continuing challenge, but it was too far ahead of events and without immediate effect on practice.

Public policy culminated in the National Health Service Acts of 1946 and 1947. Their definition of statutory boundaries between hospital and general practice, and the consequential hospital policies underlined the end of an era. On the other hand the NHS was predicated on the existence of a stalwart front line of practice. The shock of changes which it emphasized but did not create, and the needs of the new situation have set in train a continuing process of reappraisal of the position and needs of general practice. The statutes themselves contributed little to the positive definition of general practice; a point noted in 1950 by the Cohen Committee on General Practice and the Training of the General Practitioner (28):

The Committee had not proceeded very far in discussing its terms of reference before it found it necessary to define the nature of the work of the general practitioner and the aims and purpose of his post-graduate education. The Medical Acts do not help; they were framed before the present division of medical practice into special branches had far advanced. Official regulations under the National Health Insurance Act and the National Health Service Acts do not help; they speak only of 'the range of service to be rendered by a general practitioner under the Act' without further definition. Phrases such as 'the backbone of the profession' and 'the first line of defence' which are often applied to general practitioners may flatter but they lack precision. Some speak of general practice as though it comprises those minor medical responsibilities which remain after the work regarded as 'specialties' has been withdrawn; others regard the practitioner as an index to the appropriate specialist.

The process of shock treatment for general practice continued with polemics on its problems. Collings was first in the field (1).

The value of his analysis and recommendations tended to be overlooked in the affront created by his harsh criticism. He called attention to the dangers of well-intentioned but unilateral planning of hospital services. Weakness in general practice did not result in specific analysis of its needs and effort to strengthen it. The response was to substitute with hospital services, removing responsibility from general practice and so weakening it still further.

> Thus hospital and specialist requirements are being worked out with no real regard to the present state, or the future development, of general practice. I saw a good example of this when I visited two hospitals, of similar size and type, which had been included in a previous hospital survey and had lately been assessed for staff and equipment. One of them worked in association with a long-established group practice and the other in association with a number of doctors working independently. The work that was being done by the group completely altered the requirements of the first of these hospitals; yet nobody official had ever visited the group or taken any account of the things that were being done, or could be done, by it. Even in situations like this, where the whole history and development of the hospital had been in the hands of the general practitioner, the future of the hospital now seems to be considered as something apart from him. This is an extension of the attitude which has prevailed in larger hospitals for a long time—i.e. that the general practitioner has no place in hospital work and therefore merits no direct consideration in hospital planning and development.

Other visitors from overseas were unattracted by what they saw. Thus Diehl and his colleagues from the United States wrote (29):

> The general practitioner no longer has access to a hospital for patients under his care. If his patients need laboratory tests, roentgen examinations or special study for diagnosis or treatment, he must refer them to a hospital. He then has no further responsibility for the medical care of his patient since he has no privileges in the hospital. His work is limited to home calls and office visits. Payment of general practitioners is on an annual per capita basis. Therefore, in order to have an adequate income, the general practitioner tries to keep as many patients on his list as possible.
>
> The status of the general practitioner at the present time appears

to be the most crucial defect in the National Health Service. Over the past 30 years, under the original system of 'panel practice', there has developed a type of general practice which was limited largely to home and office care with some small opportunity for hospital practice. The National Health Service has extended this and has made the distinction between general practice and consultant practice in the hospital even sharper than ever.

In order to improve general practice, efforts are being made to providc general practitioners continued educational opportunities, financed by the Ministry of Health. Unfortunately, nothing has been done to make it possible for him to practise with greater competence after additional training.

Sir Heneage Ogilvie was brusque and outrageous in his comments (15):

The final and official segregation came with the National Health Service Act. After July 1948, the medical profession was split into categories, defined with the verbose exactness of the Civil Servant. Each man, after qualification, pre-registration employment and national service must enter or be herded into one of several pens, and within that pen he must live until he dies or retires. Of these pens, the lowest is that of general practice. General practice was artificially debased. The general practitioner was made a shuffler of patients' cards, a signer of certificates, a distributor of benefits, a treater of minor ailments within strictly defined limits and with strictly specified remedies, a stooge with a twenty-four hour working day, liable to be victimised by trivial complaints but forbidden to complain himself. The specialist was artificially elevated. All citizens may demand specialist treatment, therefore specialists must be turned out to fill the demand. We are now in a ridiculous position where a well-trained and competent doctor is forced to refer his patient to a man of lesser ability but marked with the correct rubber stamp, in order that he may carry out treatment that he himself could do very much better. Hospitals have accumulated unmanageable waiting-lists because their beds are blocked by patients undergoing treatment that could very well have been carried out at home, by patients admitted for investigations that the practitioner could have conducted himself had he been granted X-ray and laboratory facilities, and by patients retained merely through the fear of litigation bred by a series of legal decisions that seem to have been given on the simple working rule that the doctor is always wrong . . .

But the tide of consideration was turning. There began a series of reports and recommendations to bring support to the needs of general practice. The British Medical Association set up in series two committees under the chairmanship of Henry Cohen on *The Training of a Doctor* and on *General Practice and the Training of the General Practitioner* (28, 30).

The Cohen Committees brought a new dimension into the debate by declaring that the GP could no longer be regarded as a kind of residual doctor, but must be seen as a specialist in his own right with special needs for postgraduate education and vocational training related to his unique responsibilities and skills. The second committee also made recommendations about ways and means of supporting the work of the practitioner and associating him with the hospital. Later the Gillie Committee amplified these recommendations (31).

The difficulties remain of materially altering the specifications of general practice by changes restricted to it as an entity separate from the rest of medical care. All boundaries in a medical care system are arbitrary. Can one component be changed substantially without some realignment of the system as a whole?

McKeown has drawn attention to this issue by his suggestions (32). His recommendation that the personal doctor should specialize by age-groups is very controversial, but it is a significant token of the radical re-thinking required to permit the changes he thinks necessary to give a new future to the personal doctor; that he must work with his patients in hospital as well as outside to keep up to date and to ensure continuity of care; and there must be a shift in the division of responsibility between the personal doctor and the consultant to allow this to happen.

> Doctors who are not consultants should provide personal medical care in patients' homes, at a health centre, and in hospital. In future it will be desirable for all doctors to specialize, and since it is no longer possible for one person to maintain clinical competence in the care of all age groups the best arrangement would be to divide medical responsibility according to the age of patients. In childhood, in adult life, and after retirement the medical and related social problems are relatively homogeneous. It is therefore suggested that

a more satisfactory basis of practice would be one in which personal medical care is provided by four types of doctors: obstetrician, paediatrician, adult physician and geriatrician. This concept of the personal doctor is not inconsistent with the definition of a general practitioner suggested by the College of General Practitioners in 1957: 'A doctor in direct touch with patients, who accepts continuing responsibility for providing or arranging their general medical care, which includes the prevention and treatment of any illness or injury affecting the mind or any part of the body.'

The final quotation calls attention to the most glorious event of all in the recent story of general practice, the establishment in 1955 of the Royal College of General Practitioners. Its sustained and disinterested efforts for improvement in the work of the personal doctor suggest that once again the practitioners may lead the way to reform.

MEDICAL EDUCATION AND THE GENERAL PRACTITIONER

General practice received its highest accolade when the new General Medical Council established by the Medical Act 1858 took their specific needs as the measuring rod for a sound curriculum. Whatever later views might be, at that time it was reasonable to suppose that a clearly held view of the nature of general practice as then understood could allow an equally clear definition of the education required. On registration the practitioner stepped forth into immediate responsibility, so the coverage must not only be sufficient in scope it must also be detailed enough to ensure the safety of the public. So it was possible to hope for a perfect match between job and education. At the same time it seemed that the requirements of the embryo consultant were no different from those of the man who became a GP on qualification. The consultant could build his additional knowledge by practice on the same foundations. The objective of medical education in Britain became the production of the safe GP. Although the objective seemed clear the Council was slow to show its hand. Its powers were limited, and there were internal differences to sort out. First it set about making recommendations to raise the standard of general education for entry into medical education. By 1869 it was looking at more detailed propositions about curriculum and order of study. It was examining a proposition that it might spread its views amongst the licensing bodies by compiling a set of rules (16).

This was a forecast of the system of periodic recommendations by which the Council has made known its views on requirements for medical education to licensing bodies. Over the years the recommendations specified the needs in terms of the production of the safe practitioner, with a tendency to increasing detail of specification.

Despite the apparent ease and simplicity of the formula of the 'safe general practitioner' as the objective of medical education, the very events which had achieved reform in 1858 and the establishment of the Council held the seeds of destruction of any static definition of objectives of medical education. The impact of scientific development in medicine was one of the forces which had brought into existence the new breed of practitioners who demanded reform. It was the implications of continuing scientific development which exposed the inadequacy of the concept that in a rapidly changing world of practice any practitioner could be made safe for a lifetime of practice by his basic education at medical school. Flexner in his reports on medical education to the Carnegie Foundation already in 1910 and 1912 exposed the fallacy of the 'safe doctor' concept. Medical science was moving so fast that ideas learnt at medical school were bound to be out of date long before the practitioner had come to the end of his career. The object of medical education must be to prepare the student to keep up to date through his career by his scientific approach to medicine and his habits of learning (33).

Medicine is changing with unprecedented rapidity. It has undergone greater changes in the last three decades than in the preceding three centuries—a rate of speed likely hereafter to be accelerated, not retarded. On what terms can the physician or surgeon participate in progress? To put the same question differently: the utmost practical capacity and judgment attainable at school are in no event huge; as things now move, they are soon more or less antiquated. If a choice must be made between some portion of this positive attainment and markedly greater ability to participate in the development of medical science, which alternative should medical education prefer? To ask the question is to answer it . . . The fact is, that the rapid progress of medical science has necessarily changed the role of the medical school: a substantially stationary or slowly changing medical and surgical art could be communicated; the level did not appreciably alter in the course of a professional life-time. A boy who learned medicine at school knew it for the rest of his life. But expanding sciences and the arts dependent on them cannot be totally, even largely, imparted in a few months. The greatest service to be rendered the student is in giving him such training as will enable and incline him to keep up and to go ahead.

Later he wrote (34):

A medical school cannot expect to produce fully trained doctors, it can at most hope to equip students with a limited amount of knowledge to train them in the method and spirit of scientific medicine, and to launch them with a momentum that will make them active learners, observers, readers, thinkers and experimenters for years to come.

It was not till the General Medical Council's recommendations of 1957 and the report of the Royal Commission on Medical Education in 1968 that Flexner's views were fully expressed as public policy. Their specifications for a scientific doctor suggest the need for a new equilibrium to be established between general practice and medical education. After 1858 education was made to fit the immediate needs of practice. Perhaps this time it is the circumstances of general practice which should be altered to fit more closely the needs and aspirations of the new doctors.

The Royal Commission on Medical Education has recently stated what our educational objectives now should be.

Modern medical practice based as it is on rapidly changing scientific and technical knowledge, demands practitioners with the capacity to keep abreast of the tide. This is only possible if they are educated to think scientifically and to study and learn for themselves. The objective is in a sense the opposite of the 'safe doctor' concept. Basic medical education is only a first degree preparation for vocational training, and continuing self-education throughout life. Only in this way, we are told, can the doctor keep himself in shape to bring the benefits of modern medicine to his patients.

Perhaps the most significant thing in the report of the Royal Commission on Medical Education is what it did *not* say. The biggest question in medical education is whether we should plan to have one medical profession all of whose members are educated to the same basic scientific standards and expectations, or whether we should abandon this arrangement and divide into two or more parts, educated to different specifications. The Royal Commission was so confident of the correct answer to this question, that it did not discuss the alternatives. In this respect they came to the same decision as virtually all comparable reviews in other countries as well as our own.

It is not inevitable that this should be so, but the virtual unanimity of view suggests that there are even greater problems in the alternatives than in the chosen solution. Nevertheless the *feldscher* still exists in the USSR. Current attempts to reproduce something similar are publicized in the United States (35) and occasional voices are raised in this country to suggest that we should follow suit (36). The argument is that the volume of trivial illness to be dealt with in the NHS, does not warrant the efforts of the fully trained scientific doctor, but should be looked after by a subordinate grade of doctor, trained in a shorter time and to less-ambitious specifications. This is not the place to argue the case for or against such proposals; there is, however, good reason to suppose that adoption of the solution of the sub-doctor creates many problems, probably many more than it solves.

Another solution sometimes discussed is the creation of what might be called the clinician social worker. This is not canvassed as a short-cut, but because it is said that primary medical care requires a different kind of person from other branches of medicine; and therefore the training should be radically different, giving much more attention to cultural and psycho-social needs than the training of future hospital doctors. The Royal Commission's view was that all doctors require training and motivation towards social and psychological responsibilities, although the future GP has special needs.

The acceptibility or otherwise of the more radical suggestions depends in the last resort on our views of the tasks of the doctor, whether he works in the front line or in hospital. If he is seen to carry full diagnostic responsibilities, then the conclusion of the Royal Commission seems to follow—all doctors should be educated to similar scientific standards; although some may need greater sophistication than others in social responsibilities.

The point I want to make is not related to the merits of the decision of the Royal Commission (which I happen to believe to be the correct decision), but rather to its consequences. Concentration on the explicit aspects of our education process—in this case, all the fascinating details of curricula for undergraduate and postgraduate medical education—often blind us to the implicit aspects and consequences of the process. Medical education is not only a programme which builds knowledge and skills in its recipients; it is also an experience which creates attitudes and expectations. The informal atmosphere and influences are as important as the explicit pedagogic efforts. They create in the minds of the participants associations between the idea of good practice and the surroundings and resources in which it is carried out. They create expectations of standards of work to be achieved and problems to be solved. Such expectations may in a sense be distorted by a particular environment in which they develop, and it is often said that they are excessively affected by the circumstances that clinical education takes place almost entirely in hospital. The main influence, however, comes from the assumptions deriving from the objective of creating the scientific doctor, that he should learn how to solve his problems scientifically, and that appropriate tools and other resources are required for this job.

A scientific approach is not necessarily dependent in fact on particular apparatus or surroundings. Nevertheless a very significant effect of this education process is to build in the minds of its recipients notions about the circumstances of good practice.

They are likely to wish to be surrounded by similar circumstances and to feel deprived if they are not. The circumstances of good practice are associated in their minds with capacity for problem solving, and the resources needed for this. A strong urge is inculcated to be a 'good doctor'; self-esteem becomes related to the individual's estimation of whether he is or is not able to practice what he believes to be 'good medicine'. If he cannot, his self-rating of his work and consequently his morale may be affected, with loss of that continuing self-education which is one of the assumptions on which the scientific doctor concept is founded.

There are relativities in all these things. If the doctor is far from other resources he will usually continue to feel challenged to produce the best results with what hc has. If he is working in circumstances he believes to be deprived, alongside others who have the desirable resources, he is much more likely to downgrade his efforts in his own eyes with unfortunate consequences for his morale.

There is another aspect of the situation which warrants mention. Higher skills are in some senses more vulnerable than those of a simpler kind. They flourish through practice, but tarnish rapidly through disuse. In theory at any rate the decision to pursue an expensive educational policy of creating scientifically trained doctors should carry with it the consequential decision to create the surroundings of practice which potentiate the work and morale of the doctors created by this process.

There is evidence to suggest that some of our more serious problems stem from the fact that there is a dislocation between our educational policy and the attitudes created by it, and the service arrangements provided for a large number of the doctors produced. A major issue before us is to reconcile this dilemma. This could in theory perhaps be achieved by changing the education policy, but the die is cast, and we may not in any case wish to modify these decisions, although we might wish to modify some of the surrounding circumstances. If this is so, a real solution can only come by changing the service end of the equation; that is to say by altering the circumstances of practice of all doctors so that these provide an environment calculated to promote the professional satisfactions, self-esteem, and morale of our practitioners who have been motivated by the process of scientific medical education. Specifically the challenge before us relates largely, although not entirely, to the future requirements of general practice.

The signs and symptoms of the dislocation mentioned above have been intensified by the creation of a world market for doctors, a market which will continue to expand so long as economic prosperity continues. Many of the overt signs of difficulty show themselves in evidence deriving from emigration of doctors, but not all. There are signs which appear quite early on, in fact at the medical student stage. Only 23 per cent of the 1966 sample of final-year students canvassed for the Royal Commission expressed an intention to go into general practice. And although in the snapshot pictures taken for the Commission, more final-year students showed interest than first-year students, this was in itself possibly an indication of loss of interest of successive student cohorts, rather than a growth of enthusiasm during the education process (37).

There is a good deal of evidence that medical students and young doctors selecting themselves for general practice are increasingly recruited from the academically weaker end of the spectrum (38–9). This fact is not necessarily bad in itself, for academic performance is by no means always related to achievement in practice (40). It is, however, a significant observation, both as an indicator of student estimates of general practice as a field compatible with the aspirations created in them by their education and previous assumptions, and also because there is further evidence that the academically weaker students have less successs than their stronger brethren in achieving good postgraduate clinical training (38); and there is evidence that the quality of postgraduate training is significant in determining quality of subsequent practice (40).

John Last has shown rather neatly the service discrepancies implied by the lack of enthusiasm of students for general practice. By relating expressed intentions of students whose opinions were canvassed to subsequent career opportunities in the NHS, he indicated that whereas hospital specialties tended to be over-subscribed, sometimes heavily, general practice was under-subscribed by 50 per cent of its estimated requirements (40).

Perhaps we could tolerate this situation, if there were no open market for doctors elsewhere; but we are no longer able to disregard the ambitions of the young, because they can now seek outlets in other lands. No doubt there are many reasons why permanent emigration of our doctors seems to be running at a figure close to 20 per cent of our production, but the commonest element discovered is the young doctor with frustrated ambitions in a hospital specialty, who chooses to emigrate in the hope of obtaining hospital facilities elsewhere, rather than enter British general practice (42). The Department of Health team which visited North America to estimate the prospects of bringing British doctors back to the United Kingdom was forcibly struck by the comments of those they interviewed there who were in general practice. Universally they condemned the lack of facilities for the GP in Britain, and praised the hospital privileges available to them in North America. The virtually total verdict seemed to be, 'no return until comparable arrangements could be made here' (43). It may be thought that in more recent years since the Charter the tide of recruitment to general practice has turned in this country (44).

The fact seems to be that recent increases in numbers of principals in practice, are entirely accounted for by recruits qualified outside the United Kingdom. Our own graduates do not seem to have changed their verdict yet (45). It may be felt that there is not likely to be much change, until the circumstances of general practice itself are changed to be in line with the aspirations and assumptions of the scientific doctor. The necessary changes are considerable. They imply the creation of diagnostic facilities within the immediate workshop of every doctor; the build-up of a larger environment of clinical colleagueship and ancillary support. It is difficult to envisage such changes without major regrouping of practice, at least in the urban areas. These matters cannot be dealt with here in detail. They are mentioned only to bring out their implications for the needs and aspirations of doctors and their patients, and the relationship of education to practice.

There is another question of change at least as far-reaching. This is the question of the relationship of the GP to the hospital —not only as a member of a specialist team; but perhaps more forcibly, the question of his access to look after his own patients. Such an arrangement appears to conflict with the tidiness and efficiency of our system of closed specialist hospital staffing. It is the profession itself which must answer the question because in reality it is the hospital specialist section of the profession which can deny or permit this kind of access. At least the question must be treated seriously. There seems no doubt of the enthusiasm of practitioners who have grown accustomed to this facility. If in the process they are brought closely in contact with specialist colleagues, there is evidence to suggest an effect of increased quality of work as well as interest. The hospital has become so significant in modern medicine as the centre of stimulus that we must ask whether it is any longer appropriate to deny its facilities to a large section of the profession. There are, however, large questions to be answered. Given the circumstances of British general practice, would some incentive have to be created and if so, what, to induce existing practitioners to use hospital facilities if granted? Perhaps more important, what redeployment of resources and responsibilities will be necessary to create a new and different future for their successors?

REFERENCES

1. Collings, J. S. (1950). *Lancet*, i, 555, 567, 571.
2. Holloway, S. W. F. (1964). *History*, xlix (167), 306, 314.
3. Rivington, W. (1888). *Medical Professions of the United Kingdom* (London: Longmans), pp. 251–2, 275, 965.
4. Roberts, R. S. (1964). *Med. Hist.* 8 (3), 217–34.
5. ——— (1969). *Cent. Afr. J. Med.* 15 (9), 199–205.
6. ——— (1969). *Br. J. vener. Dis.* 45 (1), 58–60.
7. Poynter, F. N. L. (ed.) (1961). *The Evolution of Medical Practice in Britain* (London: Pitman), pp. 8–15, 49–50, 74–6.
8. Carr-Saunders, A. M., and Wilson, P. A. (1933). *The Professions* (Oxford: Clarendon Press).
9. De Styrap, J. (1890). *The Young Practitioners* (London: Lewis), p. 7.

10. NEWMAN, CHARLES (1957). *The Evolution of Medical Education in the Nineteenth Century* (London: Oxford University Press).

11. RIVINGTON, W. (1879). *The Medical Profession* (Dublin), pp. 55, 100.

12. MAPOTHER (ed.) (1868). *The Medical Profession and its Educational and Licensing Bodies*, p. 74.

13. SHAW, G. B. (1930). *The Doctor's Dilemma* (London: Constable), pp. xxv, xxxix.

14. MCCONAGHEY, R. M. S. (1966). *Jl R. Coll. Gen. Practit.* 2, 10.

15. OGILVIE, SIR H. (1953). *Br. med. J.* 2, 707–9.

16. HESELTINE, M. (1949). *Med. Press*, 222, 221, 228.

17. MCMENEMEY, W. H. (1959). *The Life and Times of Sir Charles Hastings* (Edinburgh, London: E. & S. Livingstone), pp. 337, 433.

18. STEVENS, R. (1966). *Medical Practice in Modern England* (New Haven: Yale University Press), pp. 3–4, 33, 56.

19. MACNAMARA, D. W. (1960). 'A century of general practice and after', *J. Irish med. Ass.* 46, 2.

20. HARDY, H. N. (1901). *The State of the Medical Profession in Great Britain and Ireland in 1900*, pp. 20–1.

21. MINISTRY OF HEALTH (1945). *Hospital Survey: The Hospital Services of London and the Surrounding Area*, by Gray, A. M. H., and Topping, A. (London: HMSO), p. 5.

22. BROTHERSTON, J. H. F. (1963). 'Towards new incentives', *Lancet*, i, 1119–21.

23. HADFIELD, S. J. (1953). *Br. med. J.* 2, 706.

24. HAMILTON, J. G. M. (1953). Ibid. 2, 711–14.

25. HUNT, J. H. (1961). Ibid. 2, 849.

26. NEWMAN, SIR G. (1939). *The Building of a Nation's Health* (London: Macmillan Co.), pp. 405–6.

27. MINISTRY OF HEALTH (1920). Consultative Council on Medical and Allied Services, *Interim Report on the Future Provision of Medical and Allied Services* (Dawson of Penn Report) (London: HMSO), pp. 11–13.

28. BRITISH MEDICAL ASSOCIATION (1950). *General Practice and the Training of General Practitioners* (Cohen Report) (London).

29. DIEHL, *et al.* (1950). *J. Am. med. Ass.* 143 (17), 1498–9.

30. BRITISH MEDICAL ASSOCIATION (1948). *The Training of a Doctor* (Cohen Report) (London).

31. MINISTRY OF HEALTH (1963). Standing Medical Advisory Committee, *The Field of Work of the Family Doctor* (Gillie Report) (London: HMSO).

32. MCKEOWN, T. (1965), *Medicine in Modern Society* (London: Allen and Unwin).

33. CARNEGIE FOUNDATION FOR THE ADVANCEMENT OF TEACHING (1912). *Medical Education in Europe*, by Flexner, A. (Bulletin No. 6), pp. 274–5.

34. FLEXNER, A. (1925). *Medical Education* (New York: Macmillan Co.).

35. DUKE UNIVERSITY (1969). 'Physician's assistant program, 1960–1970', *Bull. Duke Univ.* 41, 8–D.

36. HILL, K. R. (1968). *Lancet*, i, 351.

37. ROYAL COMMISSION ON MEDICAL EDUCATION (1965–8). *Report*, Cmnd 3569 (London : HMSO), pp. 145, 286, 358, 361.

38. LAST, J. M., MARTIN, F. M., and STANLEY, G. R. (1967). *Proc. R. Soc. Med.* 60, 813.

39. WHITFIELD, A. G. W. (1969). *Lancet*, i. 667.

40. PETERSON, O. L., *et al.* (1956). 'An analytical study of North Carolina General practice 1953–54', *J. Med. Educ.* 31, no. 12, part 2.

41. LAST, J. M. (1967). *Lancet*, ii, 769.

42. ABEL-SMITH, B., and GALES, K. (1964). *British Doctors at Home and Abroad* (Welwyn : Codicote Press).

43. *Br. med. J.* (1968), 1, 45.

44. REVIEW BODY ON DOCTORS' AND DENTISTS' REMUNERATION (1970). *Twelfth Report*, Cmnd 4352 (London : HMSO).

45. CARGILL, D. (1969). *Lancet*, i, 669.

Discussion

The issues concerning medical practice, and particularly the role of the primary physician, are perhaps the most important confronting medical education today. In the USA some consultants who have spent most of their professional lives in teaching hospitals have begun to question a system based on the provision of specialists for all patients' requirements. The good internist is well trained in the diagnostic and therapeutic measures of internal medicine, but he is a very expensive and inefficient purveyor of medical care. In comparison with the GP, he takes longer to examine a patient, he uses more X-ray and other costly equipment, and he spends a surprising amount of time communicating with other doctors; it is questionable whether a system based exclusively on this type of practice can meet the needs of all patients. In the USA perhaps a quarter of the population do not have an identifiable doctor, although the ratio of doctors to population is higher than in Britain. It is against this background that many Americans look with interest to British general practice, and with concern at the problems with which it is confronted.

In Britain also the trend towards specialization is evident and raises similar problems. The hospital specialist usually sees his patient at a single point in time, often for the first time, and without personal knowledge of his home and environment. With the increase in specialization few would question the need for a general physician to advise the patient and to protect him from the risks of mistaken diagnosis and treatment. This role has hitherto been filled in many cases by the GP. Why should this type of practice, highly regarded on both sides of the Atlantic, and even more necessary in future to offset the risks associated with specialization, be considered by many, including its advocates, to be in danger of extinction? If general practice is in decline, it is clearly important to try to account for it.

One influence has been the environment in which the doctor is placed. The Collings Report provided a vivid, if somewhat slanted, picture of British general practice twenty years ago, and while conditions have improved there are still too many single-handed and small partnerships, working from doctors' homes. It is also a question to what extent continuity of medical care is provided today, or indeed is attainable, particularly in the central areas of the major cities. It is on these and other grounds that some oppose the emphasis on general practice; they believe that when the patient is not seriously ill it is not important for him to be visited by a doctor in his own home, and when he is ill he will receive much better care at hospital. But although the dialogue continues between the advocates of general and specialist care, of home and hospital care, there is no doubt that the weight of opinion, medical as well as public, favours the continuation in some form of a personal medical service.

The relation of the primary doctor to the consultant and to the hospital is the central issue raised by the future of medical practice. Although the GP is often considered to be the heir of the apothecary, in the form with which we are familiar general practice began in the nineteenth century. It is largely attributable to the establishment of hospitals, which replaced the traditional divisions between physician, surgeon, and apothecary by a new one between doctors who had hospital appointments (consultants) and those who had not (GPs). It is now accepted by many, but by no means all people, that this division is unsatisfactory, and that the primary doctor should have a significant role in hospital. The identification of this role is one of the major problems confronting the medical services. An interesting investigation, one of many which will be needed, has been planned in Boston between the Beth Israel Hospital and a local community.

In Britain emphasis is rightly placed on the health centre as the main source of GP and related services in the community. This concept, outlined as early as 1920 by Lord Dawson, has only recently begun to be realized. The centres are intended to provide a basis for group practice, and it is probable that within such practices doctors will choose to specialize. It is important that this development should not be at the expense of personal and continuous medical care.

Another question, one which has had more attention in the USA than in Britain, is whether the doctor should be assisted, and in some cases possibly replaced, by a medical assistant who has had a shortened type of medical training. Experiments on these lines are in progress in the USA with the training and employment of assistants in obstetrics, paediatrics, and internal medicine. Similar experiments have been made in other countries and some of them have collapsed, for example in India and West Africa. Even if the need for this type of assistance is accepted, it remains to be seen whether it should be provided by introducing new types of health workers or by modifying in certain circumstances the role of the nurse.

In this context there are some interesting international differences in experience and outlook. Since Flexner, American medicine has aimed for quality, whereas after the Revolution Russia deliberately decided to achieve quantity. At a time when Russian medicine is becoming more concerned with quality, America is seeking to introduce analogues of the *feldscher*. In Britain dental hygienists and health visitors in general practice were unacceptable until recently, and the nurse is still not used as an anaesthestist though readily accepted in the USA. And in the USA medical and public opinion is ready to have women as obstetrical assistants, while unwilling to accept the European model of a midwife.

There are also many residual questions concerning the recruitment, undergraduate education, and postgraduate training of the doctor. There can be little doubt that the image of medicine projected at the teaching centre has a profound influence on the decisions of students concerning their future careers, and it is for this reason that many medical schools are exploring the development of departments or sub-departments concerned with general practice. Finally the survival of general practice will depend on conditions of work and remuneration, but even more on the attractiveness of the job that is assigned to the practitioner. In the postgraduate field British medicine is indebted to the Nuffield Provincial Hospitals Trust whose conference in 1965 was the point of origin of the postgraduate centres which have subsequently developed throughout the country. They are making an indispensable contribution to the continued education of the doctor and could in time lead to a revolution in general practice.

Finally, there is great need for investigation of new patterns of medical practice. In some cases this can take the form of study of innovations in practice where they exist, and the Health Insurance Plan of New York and the Kaiser-Permanente Organization provide examples of new developments which repay examination. But in addition it will be desirable to experiment with new patterns of care and to compare the experience of different patterns before deciding on models which should be widely followed. For example, in both United States and Britain it should be possible to mount experiments to investigate the organization of health centres and the role of GPs in hospital, using populations of about 200,000 as a base. The results of such experiments would be much more instructive than conclusions drawn from abstract discussions of the role of the GP. It goes almost without saying that such experiments should be the concern not only of doctors, but also of persons trained in fields such as business administration and management.

5

HISTORICAL DISCONTINUITY, HOSPITALS, AND HEALTH SERVICES

PAUL J. SANAZARO

Historical discontinuity, hospitals, and health services

INTRODUCTION

Scholars entrusted with advancing history as a discipline differ in opinion on the social uses and values of historical study. None the less, Thucydides' view persists that 'knowledge of the past is an aid to the interpretation of the future'. Recorded history is at root a succession of particulars. Some say it is proper, if not necessary, to select a current problem or situation as the retrospective frame within which to identify and interpret relevant antecedent events. The intent is to isolate and understand more clearly 'historical causes'. In a broad epidemiological sense, such may be construed as an attempt at 'preventive history': drawing on the past to highlight for us potentially undesirable and avoidable consequences of future decisions.

Traditional historians shun this 'retrogressive modernism'. They charge that imposing interpretations of contemporary institutions or political and social processes on the past may 'falsify' history. When separated from the context of their times, they say, ideas and events may mistakenly be thought to fit into a coherent historical trend when, in fact, the historian's obligation is to explain how the ideas and events fitted into the milieu of their time.

Without partisanship, this paper draws on the approaches of both schools.

Our foray into history must define the hospital as an institution in health services and in society at large. McKeown has set the stage through his concise chronicling of what is wrong with hospitals today (1). If we identify and analyse adequately the historical circumstances responsible for the present situation, he suggests, we may forestall future similar missteps and perhaps find some useful new insights.

The hospital is one component of medical care and of health services generally. It is the crossroads of the science, art, politics, and economics of medicine, but has no functions independent of advancing health services for people. Accordingly, I propose an alternative search for historical enlightenment. The object is to trace the evolution of the modern hospital, since about 1800, in the context of 'health services systems'. This retrospecting frame looks at hospital services in the perspective of progressively more explicit relationships among all the components of the health services.

My discussion embodies two themes, each derived from historical analysis. The first is that hospital services are on a plateau in their evolution while health services and their contributing sciences are in transition towards more formal systems. Leading up to the plateau are centuries of unco-ordinated, autonomous growth. Ahead is the era of interdependent planning and decision-making which will integrate all institutional and extra-institutional health services. The present situation is considered neither a culmination nor necessarily an immediate prelude.

The second theme is a paraphrase of Whitehead's notion that intellectual progress occurs in three stages. For the past twenty years, research in health services has excited us with its promises. This epitomizes the 'stage of romance'. However, the task of moving on to the 'stage of precision' remains before us. We may be able to take this step through a new form of R & D. Designed to produce working prototypes of health services components and systems, it can supply the rationality for planning and decision-making. Whitehead's third stage, generalization, is intrinsic to the design of health services R & D.

I. HISTORICAL PERSPECTIVES

To compare instructively the evolution of hospitals in our respective countries requires competence in adjusting for the great differences in our nations' ages, social philosophies, and political processes. Such is the preserve of historians. This discussion is limited mainly to the American scene, drawing upon related developments in Grcat Britain at selected historical nodal points.

Time frame 1: 1800–1920

Detailed histories of hospitals are available (2, 3, 4) and McKeown has provided the paths along which selective analyses of historical determinants must proceed:

> . . . throughout the period when most (hospitals) were built there were . . . separate authorities . . It was possible to build a hospital anywhere and for any purpose. Hospitals were founded in the most casual and sometimes irresponsible manner: by the provision of a will; by the whim of an eccentric benefactor; by the design of young physicians or surgeons to improve their prospects; by the wish of a small community to have its own hospital. In such ways was the location, size, and character of many hospitals determined with little regard for the needs of patients or for the fact that the shape of the services was being fixed for more than a century.
>
> The effects of this unplanned development were disastrous (1).

In these particulars there are more similarities than differences in our two countries. But although these two streams run parallel, others diverged early and continue to diverge: our respective patterns of organizing and financing medical care, and the social and public policies they reflect.

In the late nineteenth century, the majority of Englishmen are said to have considered free hospital care their natural right (4). Only as hospitals became necessary to apply the benefits of anaesthesia and surgery and skilled nursing care were pay-patients admitted in any appreciable numbers. In the United States, free hospital care was provided only for the destitute and in limited amounts; most beds in the late 1800s were occupied by pay-patients.

In keeping with social policy there emerged early in Britain the hospital-based physicians and, in the mid nineteenth century, organized home nursing services alongside home medical services. In the United States, such developments occurred much later and have remained modest in scope.

Since 1800, our countries have differed in providing hospital care and supporting services for the poor, in financing care, in creating organized extra-hospital services, and in separating hospital- and office-based medical practice. As a consequence, in the United Kingdom the properties of health services which connote 'system' are more evident than in the United States. This was true at the beginning of this century and remains as true today.

Despite the 'uncontrolled development' of hospitals in both nations, the amount and level of care provided in hospitals were consistent with the order and level of other social welfare services. By diverse means, society provided hospital care in amounts consistent with social policy. Although the exact curves are irregular, in their smoothed form they are, since 1800, steadily upward against the ordinates of bed/population ratios and of standards.

The ratio of hospital beds to total population is a rudimentary expression of system properties in health services. The consistency of the direction of the time series data between 1800 and 1950 means that the unco-ordinated growth of hospitals was not entirely random. However, 'unplanned' is an appropriate characterization, given today's maxim that hospital services should correspond to the population's needs.

In the last half-century, rational planning has emerged as the dominant principle guiding those concerned with organizing health services. Given this historical fact, a more detailed analysis of recent and contemporary history is in order.

Time frame 2: 1920–1970

. . . in the late 19th century the great change . . . was the invention of the method of invention. The process of change became quick, conscious, and expected. The gap was narrowed between the scientific idea and the goods and services it made possible . . .

In the first half of the 20th century the harvest of four centuries of modern science changed the aspect and outlook of our civilization as well as our daily lives and habits of thought . . . Hume in the 18th century had said that the world was more like a turnip than it was like a watch; it was now known to be more like a thought (5).

Today, only the fact and speed of societal change are unambiguous. The commonly seen signpost, 'post-industrial', directs us towards ever-increasing societal organization and interdependence, the hallmark of the current societal transition (6). The historical line tracing the evolution of hospitals and health services merges with this broader, indeed all-encompassing trend. The essence of the current history of hospitals is the beginning erosion of their autonomy.

In the United States, relatively sustained interest in hospital planning began in the 1920s, some thirty years later than in Great Britain. For the ensuing quarter-century, the underlying assumption was that appropriate geographic distribution of hospitals would bring about improvements in the delivery of care. Gradually, co-ordination of hospitals and health services was seen to be desirable. But in 1946, the monumental Hill–Burton Act was directed only to rational geographic distribution of beds. Its legislative history referred to regionalization of health services, but the law contained no specific provisions for this nor any inducements.

In the first twenty years of Hill–Burton, most construction was in areas that previously lacked a hospital or had unacceptable beds. As a consequence, distribution of physicians and nurses did improve. So did architectural and engineering design. Of special significance, Hill–Burton brought representatives of the public for the first time into the policy-making of state health departments.

There were offsets to these substantial contributions, especially the building of large numbers of small hospitals. But the intent of the Hill–Burton law was realized, even though the distribution of hospitals did not assume any regional pattern.

In the early 1950s, several voluntary area-wide planning agencies came into being. In comparing the changes which subsequently occurred in the 'planned' areas with those in 'unplanned' areas of similar characteristics, there were few differences. One reason is that planners remained largely preoccupied with hospitals and beds as isolated components.

The principle of area-wide planning became firmly established in the early 1960s when Federal funds were made available. In the mid 1960s came a profusion of new health legislation, including the Comprehensive Health Planning and Services Act of 1966. This Act and its Amendments in 1967 constitute the first national effort to institutionalize systematic health planning by creating quasi-public bodies on state and local levels. The word 'comprehensive' denotes non-categorical planning, a historical first for our country. All elements of personal and environmental health services are included. The future effects of this planning cannot yet be estimated.

1966 brought also the Regional Medical Programs legislation. This provides funds for the creation of regional co-operative arrangements among health care providers. The express purpose is to improve the care of patients suffering from heart disease, cancer, stroke, and related diseases. Fifty-five regions, covering the entire nation, are now working actively. The relationship of the Regional Medical Programs to Comprehensive Health Planning remains to be resolved.

Two recent reports in the United States are final historical proof that the system concept now dominates our views of health services. One included the following statement:

> Survey of the health systems of this Nation reveals that changes are needed and, indeed, are occurring—changes that combine planning, community responsibility, and consumer participation in a development of comprehensive health care available for all. These changes pervade all human services such as health, education, employment, transportation, welfare, urban development, and recreation. These changes refer to how these systems relate to one another and how the individual components interact within each human service system. In terms of health care, these changes raise questions about how health service systems should relate to other human

services systems, and what should be the optimal arrangements and relationships of health resources and services within the community that will deliver comprehensive health services (7).

In this apogee of our second historical time frame, the National Advisory Commission on Health Facilities explicitly related the design of the 'buildings and facilities of tomorrow' to the 'development of systems for delivery of comprehensive health care', and related these in turn to other 'human services systems'.

One year earlier, the National Advisory Commission on Health Manpower brought to an end the fruitless 'numbers game' in manpower by two forthright statements: 'The adequacy of health services depends as much upon the organization of health personnel and their combination with other resources as it does upon their numbers alone', and: *'Unless we improve the system* through which health care is provided, care will continue to become less satisfactory, even though there are massive increases in cost and in numbers of health personnel' (8).

In Great Britain, certain modifications that have been proposed in the NHS imply an emphasis on 'system':

> The removal of the present administrative barriers between the different parts of the service will enable everyone working at every level of the health service to plan, administer, and provide for the comprehensive health needs of every citizen (9).

To sum up, the earlier history of hospitals was the pre-system-concept era. The crude measure of their functioning was the ratio of beds to population, a ratio which held influence until very recently. Today there is historical discontinuity in the evolution of hospitals, reflected in the commitment to improving health services systems. Planning for hospitals and facilities and for manpower and services is seen as equalled in importance by planning for their formal interrelationships.

2. THE HOSPITAL: COMPONENT OR ORGANIZER

Hospital as a component of health services

It is appropriate to consider briefly some hospital-related data generated by health services research and its potential for influencing the likely next stages of hospital evolution.

Hospital size can be intelligently discussed only in relation to other variables (e.g., administrative, design, financial, geographic, functions) which must be prespecified. Economies of scale remain uncertain and have not been especially clarified of late. The marginal cost of an empty bed is still in dispute. A beginning has been made in validating design principles by measured improvements in staff efficiency and in realized economies of renovating.

The benefits of automated information transfer within hospitals are yet to be demonstrated beyond improving business functions, making possible higher occupancy rates, and reducing errors and delay in transmission of reports. What constitutes proper staffing in relation to changing patient mix is as uncertain today as it was ten years ago. And it remains to be proven that automation can significantly increase the efficiency of supporting services except in highly limited areas.

In the impressive mass of literature about the hospital we find little that clarifies the hospital's over-all role in health services. Surprisingly few firm answers have been given to major economic questions.

Hospital as an organizer of health services

Recurring studies of inappropriate hospital use are now well buttressed by reasonably reliable estimates of actual patient needs for institutional care. It is still said generally that suitable alternatives to hospitalization would be used willingly by the public and their physicians. Historical fact is to the contrary, however. These 'alternatives' have not been developed in the United States, despite the seemingly persuasive evidence of their need.

This stalemate is one aspect of the current debate between the 'centripetal' and the 'centrifugal' schools of thought. The former holds that the hospital is the existing organizational base capable of rationalizing the distribution of patients in accord with their actual need for institutional or ambulatory care:

> The spontaneous, voluntary efforts of many hospitals in recent years to join in such movements as accreditation, areawide planning, medical audits, utilization review, uniform accounting and pricing policies, expansion of outpatient services and extended care facilities, and joint ventures and shared services of all kinds are overwhelming evidence that the capabilities for serving as the organizing focus of a more effective health care system exists within our hospitals (10).

Wherever geographic conditions and population characteristics are favourable, such developments should be encouraged. When realized, they will provide an important opportunity for critically testing some important assumptions: that patients will benefit through more proper placement; that greater efficiency and economy of administration and operation will be realized; that long-term planning for capital expenditures can be more definitive.

The centrifugal school of thought holds that the hospital and its medical staff are oriented to acute hospital care. It observes that in-hospital services are shifting to a bimodal distribution. At one end are ever more beds for intensive care and for a new category of care between the ordinary acute and the intensive level. The other peak is the convenience admission and lengthened stay to which the public increasingly feels entitled.

Also pertinent to this side of the argument is the persisting and troubling inability to provide the aged and socially dependent individuals with appropriate types and levels of care. Despite consensus on its importance and urgency, there has emerged no generally satisfactory approach to institutionalizing a level of services somewhere between unnecessary hospitalization and inadequate home care. Responsibility for organizing this broad grey zone of long-term care has not been seized by the general hospital. Its own trends are in the opposite direction. And medical staffs cannot make professionally satisfying inroads on the conditions which comprise chronic disability in the aged.

Beyond a few unusually good examples, effective over-arching administration does not exist which can manage well both hospital services and out-of-hospital services in accord with prespecified agreements.

Hospital-based ambulatory care programmes may not provide the continuity, quality, and economies that are desired. Countries that have had experience with comprehensive hospital-based medical care centres are re-examining their position. Presumably, the hospital's philosophy of intensive pursuit of diagnosis tends to permeate all its environs. To provide adequate but not zealous multipurpose primary, preventive, and continuing care, a new generation of ambulatory care centres has been proposed by some. Designed to serve large populations, these units would be staffed by properly constituted health care teams and would rely on selected automated multiphasic health services.

The differing opinions in our respective countries regarding hospital as organizing centre or as component suggest there is sufficient merit in both points of view to warrant deliberate trials. The need is clear to establish prototypes in each category. In accord with an agreed-upon protocol, we could then prospectively analyse the major factors that bear on the utility, economy, and values of each approach.

In this brief excursion into available information and ongoing trends we have found little guidance in how to integrate hospitals and other components of health services. Had the historical trend continued in which planners focused upon number and distribution of beds as criteria that hospitals were fulfilling their appropriate function, high marks could be assured today because of sophisticated techniques now at hand. More recently, concerns have extended to include hospital size and design, size of site, and relationships among the several types of hospitals. Even given this, the available analytical methods, available data, and consensual professional judgement permit us to define the likely effective alternatives for rationalizing hospital services along such dimensions. McKeown has put forward the most comprehensive and specific plans for overcoming the undesirable effects of present-day fragmentation (1).

But against our second historical time frame, the period of beginning discontinuity, these considerations become secondary to the over-all performance of health services systems. The primary strategic issue now is how best to accelerate the evolution of health services systems within which hospitals and institutional care generally can be treated as subsystems. In keeping with these views is the recent proposal to promote the development of an integrated health service through the redefinition of functions, scope, and relationships of the district general hospital (11).

3. THE EMPIRICAL BASE FOR HEALTH SERVICES SYSTEMS

The system concept imposes the requirement to bring about and maintain functional relationships among existing components so as to assure performance in accord with specified criteria. Conceptualizing such an undertaking is an enormously complex task. It is logical to turn to theoretical modelling. Successful models would define the nature of interrelationships among hospital facilities and services and other health services. Statistics could then be collected regularly to describe the state of the system and subsystems. Current statistical surveillance of hospitals is based on limited definitions of components (beds, staff, equipment), functions (bed days, patient care, and supporting services), and salient attributes (operating costs and capital needs).

Most efforts to develop empirically based models in health services were not based on operational measures so much as implicit assumptions and beliefs regarding health care. None the less, in the past fifteen years, modelling has provided a necessary intellectual scaffolding for viewing the existing health services, and especially hospitals, within the perspective of systems. But in several critical aspects, modelling has fallen short of early expectations. It has provided few substantive re-definitions of problems. It has improved decision-making modestly. And it has yet to specify the minimum necessary information transfer within hospitals and between hospitals and other health services generally. These are the sufficiency conditions for realizing benefit from modelling (6). However, the shortcomings may not reside so much in modelling as in the 'serious lack of the consistent and comprehensive statistical information that is required for rational analysis and planning, despite a surfeit of numbers about health' (8).

To translate the concept of hospital as subsystem into operational terms, the health service system must be empirically defined. For almost a decade record linkage has been the anticipated mechanism for capturing in data the interrelationships among natural history of illness, type and location of health services received, and relevant social, economic, and environmental factors. Progress has been slow, and it will be some years before operating health services data systems can provide such information (12).

System effects versus population effects

Lacking present capability for such prospective studies, we none the less can distinguish between effects attributable to how health services are organized (i.e., system variables) and the effects of population variables (13–15). Cross-national studies based on these techniques have shown that the rate of rise in aggregate hospital expenditures is independent of the national system of care; that hospital use bears a direct relationship to availability of beds and the absence of economic barriers; that perception of ill-health is a useful proxy measure for need when distribution of services is a concern. These are skimpy foundations upon which to build new conceptual towers. But they serve vitally useful purposes in both policy and operating decision-making. The measure of health services research today is its ability to define additional general principles. The simple aggregation of even the most elegant basic studies will not in the near future help resolve the special problem of how best to relate institutional to extra-institutional health services. But such studies remain our only source of new formulations of health maintenance.

4. THE NEW ARENAS OF DECISION-MAKING

The emergence of planning committees in the twentieth century signals the institutionalization of provisional mechanisms for the more rational direction of health services. So great are the rising hopes for planning that in the United States some would assign legal powers to the voluntary planning groups to assure implementation of their recommendations (10). This may be premature, given the limited state of the art in organizing services to assure their effective and efficient distribution and direction. However, some naturally occurring experiments in franchising in the United States will shortly enable us to document the nature and extent of the objective benefits of legally enforced planning.

In the twentieth century, most health care professionals have come to understand that more formal organization is necessary to deal with the fragmentation and specialization in health services. But intellectual appreciation of the need for greater interdependence among previously separate spheres of interest is not the same as actually creating operating relationships among previously independent entities.

The hospital in microcosm illustrates the profusion of subdivisions and subspecializations internally and of interdependencies externally. From the fifteenth century well into the twentieth century, the hospital required only the services of a superintendent. Today, hospitals require an executive vice-president or president, titles which more adequately connote the vastly more complex responsibilities and functions.

Bringing about necessary 'formal organization' in a pluralistic society presents the deepest practical challenges as we seek to improve our health services systems.

The new voice in decision-making

A most stimulating recent development is the extension of consumerism into health services. Here the consumer's new role is historically unique (16). In part because of the growing public investment in health services in the United States, and in part because of the re-emergence of participatory democracy as a social theme, the public is beginning to expect the same assurances in health services as have been traditional in respect of ordinary goods and services. These developments are reinforcing the professions' commitment to assure quality through comprehensive peer review. As a result, performance accounting in medical services, especially in hospitals but also in the office, will become much more explicit and objective.

Consumer representation on policy and decision-making bodies of individual institutions, community boards, and even politically appointed bodies introduces major new legal questions. The participation of ordinary citizens in decisions that affect type and quality of services to be offered to themselves and their neighbours signals a fundamental turning point in the historical role of the health professions *vis-à-vis* the public. In the United States, 51 per cent of the members of the statewide comprehensive health planning boards must be consumers. In current discussions in England, the upward revised number of area boards appears to reflect some greater commitment to participation in decision-making by local people who are being served.

The new era of consumerism brings potential for conflicts of values. Rational planning of health services connotes greater reliance on demonstrable cause and effect rather than mere judgement and inference. Increasingly the question is raised whether medical care contributes to health status to an extent warranting the current levels of investment and expenditure. This 'care *vs* cure' dialogue may become a chronic debate as non-professionals in health services increasingly influence, directly, local allocations for office and hospital medical care; preventive health services; rehabilitative services; mental health services; institutional care for the chronically disabled; welfare services; educational programmes; environmental control measures; improvement of housing; and so on. If rational planning means implementation of professional judgements regarding the application of scientifically based knowledge in accord with socially acceptable values, the health care professional and the public may do well in their new joint planning responsibilities. If decisions increasingly turn on estimates of cost-benefit, we may see considerable turbulence when economic logic contends with the divergence between the values of a self-indulging society and scientific evidence of health services efficacy.

5. THE RATIONALE OF HEALTH SERVICES R & D

This chapter has so far presented a selective view of historical and social factors influencing hospitals and health services generally. Broad societal trends and specific developments in health services are seen as supporting a conclusion that hospitals are temporarily arrested in their evolution while health services are evolving into systems. So far, attempts to speed the creation of formal systems have had to rely on data derived from health services research. The assumed utility of such data has not been borne out by experience.

The common view is that health services research contributes to understanding of health services just as other scientific research has been productive in unlocking the secrets of nature. That a fundamental distinction exists between productive health services research and research in physical systems has been recognized by some (17). Stated oversimply, the social equivalent of a physical (i.e., deterministic) system must be created by political, legal, economic, and administrative decisions in accord with social and public policy. In health services, the additional requirement is that the system be designed to serve its multiple health-related purposes. These are requirements for assuring sufficient stability to make research in the delivery of health services productive in the same sense that the physical sciences are productive. Such stability is rare in this era of transition.

Progress in our present time frame will require a new order of engagement. At issue is the ability of the aggregate decision-making mechanisms provisionally to predetermine the likely future system states for health services, including hospitals. Also at issue is the capability of R & D to mount large-scale experiments of integrated health services systems (8).

The present barrier to more rapid development of health

services systems may be visualized as the disparity between the power of the guiding concepts in health services and the limited capabilities of the tools so far available to implement them. To mix a metaphor, the conceptual designs for health services systems, like Leonardo's plans for a flying-machine, have antedated the discovery or creation of the necessary structural materials. As measured against a landmark publication, there has been little advance in the past decade (17). This in no way impugns the validity of the concepts. The methods selected to test them were often directed to highly specific areas and the resulting data were too reductionistic for the intended purposes. It is very much as though biochemistry had preceded morbid anatomy in the evolution of medical sciences. Physicians treating patients in the sixteenth century would not have been helped by data on the blood's constituents, considering they did not yet know the structure and functions of the body's interrelated systems.

Central to the strategy of health services R & D is matching the outputs of the many decision-makers to the design and development of missing but essential elements in the organization and delivery of health services. In turn, the size and scope of these elements must be matched to the scale of the health services enterprise.

The strategy and the process of health services R & D combine system concepts, interests of the public and responsibilities of professions, guidance by national policy, and data and technical methods provided by cumulative health services research. In contrast to health services research, R & D is directed to the attainment of prespecified operational criteria. Behind the selection and design of projects and the methods of implementation is the basic rationale: the resulting health services components will constitute the supporting structures which give substance to the system principle. These supporting and mutually reinforcing elements must be developed and put into place simultaneously, the prespecified operational criteria serving as objective indicators of needed adjustments or modifications in the R & D design and implementation.

In the R & D programme of the National Center, the following is a provisional definition of the minimal elements of a health services delivery system:

(*a*) Explicit performance criteria covering access to and utilization of services (especially persons not now receiving adequate services); containment of units costs and aggregate expenditures; and assessment of effectiveness of services.

(*b*) Specified type, scope, and duration of medical and related health services to be provided, including preventive, curative, rehabilitative, and health maintenance services to all people or to major groupings.

(*c*) A geographically defined population to be served which is identified individually and by place of residence, and which is sufficiently large to require the full range of specified health services and to provide an adequate financial base for the system.

(*d*) Availability of or capability to acquire resources of professional and related manpower, facilities, and finances adequate for the specified services to the defined population.

(*e*) Arrangements for payment for services to the defined population, and for capital costs of required facilities and major equipment.

(*f*) An identified institution, agency, or corporate body which is legally accountable for continuing management and development of the system on the basis of an operational health services data system.

Health services data for management purposes is essential. It must define requirements for care by locally acceptable population surveys which are technically and financially feasible. Also to be included are samplings of hospital- and office-based content and procedures of professional practice and uniform hospital discharge data that can be related to costs and to other utilization data. Another major input is to be obtained from nationally applied protocols which address salient questions when evaluating new types of health manpower or technology, designing new inter-institutional arrangements or financing mechanisms, or introducing other large-scale developmental innovations.

In its diverse, pluralistic approaches to improving health services, the United States is now grappling earnestly with the difficulty of assuring equity of access. The United Kingdom has solved this problem in its own way. Adequate access is the first-level measure of adequate system performance. Once access is assured, R & D can proceed systematically, using current prototypes and experimental methods, to relate source, content, and site of services to population requirements. At this level, the respective contributions of hospitals and other institutions can begin to be objectively analysed. The third-level measure of system performance is the impact of health services on health status. Performance accounting now is largely limited to the first and is only done experimentally on the second level. Attainment of third-level measures faces no intrinsic theoretical, technological, or financial barriers.

Fascination with the potential benefits of a system should not blur the fact that what is actually wanted is predictability and dependability of performance, i.e., attainment of system properties, not rigid conformity with one or another paradigm. The R & D approach as described constitutes one of the sufficiency conditions for the attainment of system properties in the delivery of care. Systems will emerge to the extent such properties can be developed, maintained, and successively aggregated. It is probable that important gains can be made without developing complete and formal health services systems.

In our view, tightening up performance in health services in this manner is prerequisite to increasing effectiveness of the hospital subsystem. There is now no better answer to the hospital's future than consensual wisdom (10, 11). In this period of transition in health services, we should continue to invest in attempts to create hospitals which function as adaptable system units. Given our present inability to stipulate desired alternate performance characteristics, and given the many uncertainties in our knowledge which can only be resolved by systematic studies, it appears essential that hospitals be given maximum feasible creative guidance. The key to success in this approach is that long-sought cadre of administrators and managers trained as deliberate innovators, capable of engendering necessary public and professional acceptability. The collective impact of such men is one of the sufficiency conditions for reshaping hospitals and their services to contribute more substantially to the improvement of health services.

Intellectual excursions into the past and speculations about the future often stimulate the exhortatory centres of man. My position on R & D in health services has been stated precisely in another context:

> The concepts and tools for developing an anticipatory strategy are still being worked out . . . The methods are being tried with varying degrees of success in both the private and the public sector. The difficulties are enormous. The promise is great. The length of time and the efforts to arrive at such a strategy, and the degree of success we will attain are indeterminate. Yet, we seem to be committing ourselves to trying it (18).

SUMMARY

The evolution of hospitals since 1800 in Great Britain and the United States has been viewed in relation to the emergence of the 'system' concept in health services. Throughout the nineteenth and early part of the twentieth century, the ratio of beds to population was considered an adequate measure of hospital services. In keeping with the general societal trend towards greater interdependency, rational planning has now been institutionalized and health services are explicitly formulated as 'systems'. As a result, both conceptually and operationally, hospitals are on an evolutionary plateau while health services are in transition, becoming more formally defined systems. This is the historical discontinuity with respect to hospitals: They are no longer generally autonomatous.

Health services research can not yet clarify likely future alternatives in hospital services. Equally persuasive arguments can be made for the hospital serving as the organizational base for community health services or simply as one component among many under some form of over-all management. Modelling has not been especially helpful beyond providing essential intellectual scaffoldings. This is attributable to the lack of sufficient empirical data on health services. Record linkage still is years away as a source of such data. However, comparative cross-national studies are beginning to distinguish system effects and population effects.

Decision-making in health services is becoming complex. Collective decision-making at many different levels in the professions and in government is in itself difficult. In the foreseeable future, the public as consumer will also have a voice.

Given the maldistribution of services and the uneven access and utilization in the United States, a programme of health services R & D has been developed to attack these problems directly. Its function is to produce working prototypes of better health services components and systems. R & D combines system concepts, public and professional interests and decision-making, national policy guidance, and data and methods provided by health services research. In the United States, system performance must first demonstrate equitable distribution like that in Great Britain. Then the respective contribution of hospitals and other institutional services can be objectively analysed.

In this period of transition, hospitals and health services in general require the creative guidance of innovative administrators and managers. Their contributions and guidance are necessary to our anticipatory strategy for the future direction of health services.

REFERENCES

1. McKeown, T. (1966). *Medicine in Modern Society. Medical Planning based on Evaluation of Medical Achievement* (New York: Hafner).
2. Abel-Smith, B. (1964). *The Hospitals 1800–1948. A Study in Social Administration in England and Wales* (London: Heinemann).
3. Commission on Hospital Care (1947). *Hospital Care in the United States* (New York: Commonwealth).
4. Burdett, H. C. (1893). *Hospitals and Asylums of the World*, vol. 3 (London: J. and A. Churchill).
5. Smellie, K. B. (1962). *Great Britain since 1688* (Ann Arbor: University of Michigan).

6. Bauer, R. A. (ed.) (1966). *Social Indicators* (Cambridge: MIT Press).

7. U.S. Department of Health, Education, and Welfare (1968). *National Advisory Commission on Health Facilities. A Report to the President* (Washington, D.C.: U.S. Government Printing Office).

8. *Report of the National Advisory Commission on Health Manpower* (1967). (Washington, D.C.: U.S. Government Printing Office).

9. Department of Health and Social Security (1970). *The Future Structure of the National Health Service* (London: HMSO).

10. U.S. Department of Health, Education, and Welfare (1968). *Report of Secretary's Advisory Committee on Hospital Effectiveness* (Washington, D.C.: U.S. Government Printing Office).

11. Department of Health and Social Security. Welsh Office (1969). *The Functions of the District General Hospital* (London: HMSO).

12. Murnaghan, J. H., and White, K. L. (1970). 'Hospital Discharge Data. Report of the Conference on Hospital Discharge Abstracts Systems', Supplement to *Med. Care*, 8, 1–215.

13. Andersen, R., Smedby, B., and Anderson, O. W. (1970). *Medical Care in Use in Sweden and the United States—A Comparative Analysis of Systems and Behavior*, Research Series 27 (Chicago: Center for Health Administration Studies).

14. Kalimo, E. (1969). *Determinants of Medical Care Utilization* (Helsinki: Research Institute for Social Security).

15. Roemer, M. I. (1969). *The Organization of Medical Care under Social Security. A Study based on the Experience of Eight Countries* (Geneva: Presses Centrales Lausanne SA).

16. *Report of the Task Force on Medicaid and Related Programs* (1970). (Washington, D.C.: U.S. Government Printing Office).

17. *Towards a Measure of Medical Care. Operational Research in the Health Services. A Symposium* (1962). (London: Oxford University Press for the Nuffield Provincial Hospitals Trust).

18. National Goals Research Staff (1970). *Toward Balanced Growth: Quantity with Quality* (Washington, D.C.: US Government Printing Office).

Discussion

In spite of limitations imposed by finance in Britain since 1948, there have been great improvements in health services in general and hospital services in particular. For example, until 1925 it was said that the only knowledge London had of paediatrics was Dr Still's phone number; there were no full-time paediatricians outside the universities before the Second World War and large areas of the country had none at all. In North Wales, with a population of half a million, there was no consultant physician and only one consultant surgeon. Most anaesthetists were GPs without specialist training. An improvement in the number and distribution of specialists has been one of the most remarkable achievements of the NHS. In the same period there has also been an upgrading in hospital services throughout the country, with the result that patients are now as well cared for in non-teaching as in teaching hospitals. The two main reasons for these advances have been the remuneration of doctors by public funds and an investment in hospitals which, while it has not permitted much new building, has been sufficient to bring about a vast improvement in the quality of service.

In the USA it may be said without exaggeration that health services have reached a crisis. Although this crisis has been developing at least since the beginning of the century, it is only during recent years, and particularly since the passing of the Medicare and Medicaid legislation, that public and medical opinion has become acutely aware of it. Many influences have contributed.

An important influence has been the rapid modernization of what was until recently a cottage industry. This process has been conspicuous in hospitals which have had to adapt rapidly to the introduction of technology developed initially in other applied fields. This trend has been associated with many of the manifestations of industrialization, such as the unionization of hospital employees and the introduction of business methods of finance and management. Indeed to do full justice to these trends it would be necessary to amend the theme of this Symposium to 'History and Medical Care', in order to see developments in health services in relation to the experience of other fields. For example, present government policy in the USA favours mixed public and private management of services, and this is evident in other public institutions such as the

Post Office Department and Education as well as Health. Its critics would say that this represents an abdication of government responsibilities whereas its supporters regard it as a logical adaptation of free enterprise.

In this context an important difference between the approaches of the two countries should be noted. That of the USA is resource orientated, investment being put into systems which it is hoped will produce the desired results. In Britain interventions are in general government based, leading to the creation of agencies with responsibility for the organization of services. In the USA the difficulties have been increased by the rapid evolution of the systems approach, and in many cases the results are by no means commensurate with the investment.

Most problems now confronting hospitals in the USA had their origins in an earlier period. Proprietary hospitals have almost disappeared but many contemporary hospitals developed as private non-profit institutions, supported by religious and other groups. With the best of motives, these organizations nevertheless had very parochial interests, which they promoted without reference to general consideration of hospital needs. One of the strengths of private control of American hospitals has also been a source of weakness, for while it led to the creation of some institutions which were individually excellent, it excluded the possibility of comprehensive planning. It has also been responsible for the large number of small hospitals; many of the acute general hospitals have less than fifty beds. Yet another consequence has been a substantial duplication of services which contributes to the increased cost of medical care. For example it has become almost a status symbol for a hospital to have a cobalt unit, and the number of units has probably outstripped the supply of professionals equipped to use them. The same point can be illustrated by reference to open heart surgery; it is concentrated in a few hospitals which do it well, but a number of others maintain elaborate and expensive programmes whose standards are considerably lower.

But while many difficulties confronting hospitals can be traced to an earlier period, they have been aggravated by recent trends. Until the turn of the century hospitals did not contribute significantly to health, and patients were frequently admitted in terminal illness. It has been said that it was not until 1910 that a patient in the USA with a random disease seeing a physician at random had better than a 50 per cent chance of benefiting from the encounter. In the past twenty or thirty years the situation has changed dramatically, largely as a result of the impact of biomedical research. This has led to a change in public attitudes; people now consider health to be a right rather than a privilege and this inevitably leads to expectation of health care.

Another important influence has been the finance of medical care by insurance. This method has actually increased costs, for many policies provide benefits only when the patient is in hospital. Hence physicians often admit patients who could equally well be treated as out-patients. The advantages of comprehensive prepayment, unaffected by hospital care, are well illustrated by the Kaiser-Permanente system, where bed utilization is about half of that in the country as a whole.

During the past few years attempts have been made to introduce regional planning. In view of the great diversity of circumstances in different parts of the USA, it is most unlikely that there can be any single or simple model of health services which will be generally applicable. For example, while it would be agreed that there is need for much greater emphasis on ambulatory care, its organization will undoubtedly be quite different in different areas. In some cases it may be suitable to provide services from the hospital; elsewhere, and particularly in large sprawling cities such as Los Angeles, services will have to be offered from peripheral facilities much closer to the homes of patients if they are to be used effectively. Thus the differences—between urban and rural areas, between cities, between the affluent and depressed areas of the same city—make it most unlikely that health services can achieve the homogeneous form which may be attainable in countries such as the Netherlands and Britain.

It is now well recognized that because of its impact on the outlook of health workers in training, the role of the teaching hospital is crucial to the development of medical services. However, most teaching hospitals have stood aloof from the problems of health systems. In Britain under the NHS each region was intended to be influenced by a teaching hospital and medical school but it is only recently that this influence became significant.

Opinions differ about the steps which should be taken by teaching hospitals in order to extend their role and even about the effectiveness of the measures which have already been taken. The teaching centres of London and New York are often quoted as prototypes of the acute hospital divorced from large areas of health service, yet many of them have accepted in principle the concept of comprehensive service to a defined population and some would claim to have achieved it.

With due regard for these differences of opinion, there is no doubt that the role and control of the hospital, including the teaching hospital, is changing. In the USA some major teaching hospitals were founded on European models, and for nearly a hundred years their patients were drawn wholly from the poorer sections of the community. It was not until the end of the nineteenth century that private patients were admitted under the care of individual physicians, and this led to a mixed system. Today the trend is towards a single hospital system, but of a type quite different from that which prevailed in the early period. The non-profit voluntary institution is now heavily subsidized by government funds, through programmes such as Medicare and Medicaid, and most of the rest of the finance is derived from insurance. Having regard to the source of support of most hospitals, the form of their administration is today an anachronism.

It is also important to recognize the extent to which the hospital has become the hub of health-care systems, at least in large urban areas. This trend has its critics, who identify the hospital with the increase in specialization and the loss of personal care traditionally provided by the GP. Attempts are being made to restore the balance by creation of departments of family medicine in medical schools and teaching hospitals. This proposal was initially opposed by the American Medical Association which has now, largely, withdrawn its objections.

There has been some resistance in teaching centres to the introduction of departments of general practice, and indeed to the whole concept of enlargement of their traditional responsibilities. In part this opposition may derive from the acute shortage of physicians which has existed since the time of the Flexner Report. The past thirty years have provided clinicians with powerful tools, and it is a matter of legitimate concern that they should be in the hands of doctors trained to use them properly. This leads to an apparent antithesis between numbers and quality of doctors in training. However difficult to achieve, the aim must be to increase the supply of physicians while preserving the standards which have hitherto been established.

6

THE INFLUENCE OF MEDICAL TECHNOLOGY ON MEDICAL SERVICES

BERNARD TOWERS

The influence of medical technology on medical services

I propose to be deliberately provocative in this chapter, in the hope of sharpening up the cutting edges of a very important debate about what constitutes good patient care over a wide spectrum of 'diseases'. It is obvious enough that anyone suffering from, say, anomalous embryological development of the heart, or from some types of renal failure, from carcinoma in a reasonably early stage, or from a host of other clearly defined pathological states, is likely to live a longer and happier life if he receives the benefit of treatment by skilled medical technologists with specialist knowledge of his condition. Such treatment is possible only in highly sophisticated centres of scientific or technological excellence. As a practising scientist I should like to see such scientific centres of excellence established in such numbers that anyone whose condition warrants admission and treatment would be able to receive it. What is very doubtful, to my mind, in the current practice of clinical medicine, is the assumption or hope that *all* hospitals should aim to be of this kind. It will be argued, therefore, that the indoctrination of medical students with the supposedly overriding importance of technological methods (many of them based on a somewhat limited, naïve, mechanistic view of the human body in health and disease), has had the effect of producing too large a proportion of 'scientoid' doctors, who use potent and dangerous methods without a proper understanding of the risks involved. A distinguished professor of physics once said to me that the only reason for the success of classical physics is that it is basically so very simple. He added that he was utterly taken aback at the thought of the complexity of biological systems. One does not often come across modern, technologically minded clinicians who reflect at that level, or who illustrate the humility which such reflection must necessarily induce. Those of us in the profession whose work is orientated more towards scientifically controlled experiments in the laboratories, rather than towards clinical diagnosis and treatment, are often appalled at the evident risks that are run in modern hospital wards; appalled not only on account of the possible damage suffered by patients, but also, more immediately, by the intellectual inadequacies displayed by some of those who are prepared to take the risks. This chapter will criticize, therefore, the prevalent view that if, as yet, one cannot say that 'all's for the best in the best of all possible worlds' in modern hospital practice, 'at least it is on its way there'. It is to be expected that practising hospital clinicians will spring to the defence of their art-forms, and it might be hoped that out of the resultant discussion some valid way forward will be found, that will lead us beyond the pseudo-antithesis between medical technology and patient care.

It is well, perhaps, at the start, to recognize that traditionally and in fact, medicine is essentially an art-form or *technē*. Medical technology *is* medicine. Words have a curious habit, though, in history, of changing and interchanging their meanings. The Greek word *technē* no longer carries, in intellectual circles, the laudatory overtones that it once did. Thus today it is commonplace for academics to distinguish 'pure science' from 'mere technology' (or, by implication 'impure science'), and to distribute praise and blame in the way the adjectives in those expressions suggest. Now it may well be, as was hinted above, that in recent decades the growth of a particular type of medical technology, within an over-all mechanistic philosophy, has given rise to what appears to many to be a somewhat inhuman, cold, uncaring (in the sense of real involvement with the patient) kind of medical service. But the practice of technique as such need not by any means be accompanied by lack of care, and it clearly was not so traditionally. It may be remembered how Fielding Garrison, in the peroration on ethics to his famous history of medicine (1) quotes a part of the Sixth Precept of Hippocrates as: 'wherever the art of medicine is loved, there also is love for humanity'. Actually, Garrison strained the text here by inverting the order of words, and made a very broad generalization out of a passage which actually deals with whether or not a doctor should charge an impoverished patient. The Greek has *én gar paré philanthropie, paresti kai philotechniē*, and is better rendered as 'for where there is love of man, there is also love of the art (of medicine)'. Whichever way round it is put, of course, the correlation, at any rate, is clear. Improvements in medical technology ought always to go hand in hand with improvements in medical services or 'patient care', which is what medical services in the best sense are *for*.

One doubts, sometimes, whether or not it is the health and happiness of others (which is what anyone imbued with *philanthropiē* would wish for his fellows) that many of our most earnest and dedicated technocrats of medicine today are primarily concerned to promote. I personally will never forget the anxiety I felt when watching, on television, the smiling face of Mr Washkansky, the first of the South African cardiac transplant patients. There he was, cracking his boiled egg and joking with the nurses; telling the crowding camera team how well he felt with his 'new' heart (as indeed he surely did, with the initial relief from chronic breathlessness); praising for all he was worth the medical services he was getting. And yet to anyone who had any biological insight, any knowledge of the inevitable tensions that had been created in his body, here was a man with only two possibilities ahead of him, both of them involving an early death: either his new heart would be rapidly rejected by the body's immunological mechanisms, or else those mechanisms, including defence against infection, had been eliminated before the operation. In that more likely case, here was a totally defenceless man, being paraded and exposed for publicity purposes, beseiged on all sides by crowds of people and their attendant micro-organisms. His death sentence was already made out, and yet there he was, laughing and joking, pathetically secure in his trust in the modern experts in medical technology. Where now was the Hippocratic precept, that supposed equation we noted between love of man and love of the medical art? Where really was 'love' for Mr Washkansky, where was the real understanding, the *caring*, that he had a right to expect? Let us remember that this was no isolated example, even though it was the first: other cases followed it quickly enough, all over the world wherever the technical facilities for the simple transplant of hearts (a much less sophisticated operation than many others in the field of heart surgery) were available. Daily we followed, in press and television, macabre accounts of sick and dying people being rushed in and out of operating theatres for splenectomy and blood transfusion, bowel resection, dialysis for kidney disease, artificial respiration, and all the other life-saving (or, in these and countless other cases, 'death-prolonging') techniques now available. The last days of some of these patients must have been spent in the very depths of pain, humiliation, and despair. And yet both *philanthropiē* and *philotechniē* require, as first essentials, respect for human dignity, whether in the living or in the dying process, and a basic concern for human justice.

Patients who get into the grip, or on to the treadmill, of a modern, fully equipped and technically advanced hospital, are liable, it seems to me, to be made to suffer all kinds of indignities, and worse—I mean suffer actual harm—before they are 'released' in one way or another. And yet one of the traditional precepts of the medical profession was *primum non nocere* ('first, do no harm'). That is in no sense a precept to do nothing: what theologians call the 'sins of omission' are more insidious, more 'evil' in a sense, than are the 'sins of commission'. One can kill a patient by standing idly by. Society calls it 'criminal neglect', and may institute legal proceedings. We should also be looking at some of the positive acts (done in the name of technological advance) that might involve 'neglect'. The prescription *primum non nocere* is clearly impossible of 100 per cent attainment, even with the best will in the world. The old phrase about doctors always being able to 'bury their mistakes' recognizes this evident truth. No one can hope always to be right, and never to do harm. When one considers the current increase in complexity and sophistication of medical techniques, the question is not merely whether or not the incidence of iatrogenic morbidity and indeed mortality is on the increase: the answer to that question must surely be 'yes' in absolute figures. After all, many more people are being investigated, and treated, with successive batteries of techniques, and each of them carries with it a risk, as every interference with biological processes must of necessity do. It might be suggested that the evident advantages to those who successfully survive the experience of modern medical technology, without harmful side-effects, and in a generally improved state of health and happiness, clearly outweigh the disadvantages suffered by those who do not. And yet it is at least arguable that one should never allow even one person unwillingly to suffer for the benefit of others. It is pertinent to ask oneself whether a single case of iatrogenic disease or death, resulting directly from the careless use (misuse) of one or more of the powerful tools of modern technology, is not enough to make us pause, at least, in our current, blind admiration for technological sophistication.

Now, of course, iatrogenic disease is no newcomer in the history of medicine. *Primum non nocere* assumes its existence. In the post-mortem room in the University of Cambridge there is an inscription fixed to the wall opposite the gallery, a place where students and attending physicians cannot fail to see it. It is a remark attributed to Napoleon: 'I do not want two diseases, one Nature made and one Doctor made.' The university morbid anatomist had it placed there, not very long ago, because experience had taught him that modern clinicians need to be constantly reminded (for the safety of their patients) of the death-dealing powers they now wield. It is the pathologist who is called upon, in fatal cases of iatrogenic disease, to assess the errors or stupidities of his clinical colleagues. Sometimes his conscience may require him to criticize them publicly in the coroner's court, though much that could sometimes be said on such occasions undoubtedly goes unsaid, for obvious and not necessarily unworthy reasons. Good pathologists, who recognize only too well the particular sequence of technical errors (in medical and surgical diagnosis and treatment) that conducted the case to the post-mortem table, are under considerable social pressure to keep their own counsel, or at most to report privately and by word of mouth to the attendant clinician. It seems that they are rarely thanked for their pains: some doctors, having made a mistake, really do prefer to bury it. In the absence of written documentation (since so much, in these areas, is communicated by the spoken word), it is difficult to make a judgement about the extent of the deleterious effects on medical care (medical services) of recent, rapid increases in both sophistication and application of medical technology. But this is surely such a vital area of concern, that it calls for a confidential analysis in depth, to discover the full facts about 'failures' in current practice.

My own impression of medical students of today is that they are increasingly impressed with the sheer 'cleverness' of modern technology. Many of the techniques employed seem particularly 'sound' to our scientifically trained students (trained at least to the Advanced Level of the General Certificate of Education), because they are often so uncompromisingly numerical in nature. In the modern world a number carries with it an aura of objectivity that a mere word cannot hope to match. Also, modern medical techniques tend to isolate (as indeed they must) just a very few variables at a time, so that the numerical print-outs that come back from the laboratory, to be spread out over the patient's bed in the ward (effectively hiding him from view at times!), acquire the kind of validity that we associate more with the 'exact' sciences of physics and chemistry than with the 'inexact' science of medicine. Indeed the emphasis on 'number', in virtually all clinical reports these days, is an indication of the extent to which physics, the science of the 'very simple' (to quote again one of its modern leaders) has been adopted by medicine as the paradigm of good science. But let us also remember that biology has been called 'the science of the infinitely complex', and that medicine constitutes the most complex part of biology.

Most modern techniques of medical practice deal with some specialized, or limited, aspect or part of the organism. Each specialized technique is set in the framework of a relatively simple, or simplistic, mechanical philosophy of structure–function relationships more suitable to the nineteenth than to the twenty-first century. It inevitably follows that, for the moment at least, the student (and his teacher) sees the patient less and less as a person, more or less integrated and 'whole', and more and more as a somewhat fragmented collection of thousands of variables. Since variables are normally studied in very small groups, their over-all interdependence may entirely escape notice, because it is too complex for normal rational analysis. Alienation, at the 'human' level, is then inevitable. Some clinicians have recognized that patients may suffer harmful psychological effects if their major contacts with the profession in hospital are with doctors who spend most of their time 'with' them actually poring over the accumulated figures in the case-notes. It has been suggested that each clinical firm should have on it a social psychologist to provide what medical specialists no longer do. The psychologist would act as a counsellor, a human intermediary or point of reference and stability, between the person of the patient and the machines that his doctors not only increasingly depend on, but of which they have themselves, by a curious reversal of evolutionary development, become some kind of extension.

I think there can be little doubt that many patients resent the current obsession with technical procedures. They do so most of all when they suspect that the interest being served is not by any means necessarily their own. When patients begin to think that the doctor may be using the investigations, that they themselves are being asked or made to suffer, primarily for his own research interests, or those of the institute or department, university or country to which he belongs, then resentment can become profound. This is the more so when they feel, as they so often do, quite powerless in face of the bureaucracy of the system. English patients are very tolerant on the whole, and they have a fund of goodwill towards the medical profession. But their co-operation can easily, and rightly, be jeopardized if techniques are employed, without any evident benefit to the subject (or should it be 'object'?), which either cause pain, or are unduly time-consuming, or carry with them anything more than the minimal risk associated with every interference with biological processes. It should not go unnoticed (and I have it on excellent authority, from former preclinical pupils of mine who know they have nothing either to lose or fear by speaking frankly with me—as they might have if they dared to speak out in clinical circles) that patients in London hospitals not infrequently plead with the junior doctors (who are the ones they feel they 'know' better) not to be sent, or sent back, to a research unit where technical procedures are constant and unremitting, even though they know that the 'best brains' and the most advanced treatment for their condition might be found there.

The social and ethical dangers of 'experimental medicine' have long been recognized, and steps have been taken in more responsible centres to minimize abuses that might result from an over-enthusiastic experimentalist taking unjustifiable liberties with his 'experimental animals' in the wards. The 1964 Declaration of Helsinki, concerning the ethics of clinical research, laid down a number of principles, which local 'ethical committees' now try to see are adhered to in any projected investigation that comes to their notice. One aspect was never touched on, however, in the Declaration of Helsinki. The 1968 Bossey Conference on 'Experimentation on Human Beings' suggested many improvements, and made good this particular deficiency with the addition of a new section, entitled 'The Development and Promotion of Responsible Attitudes'. The first paragraph boldly states that 'Medical Schools, universities, and teachers should ensure that every future doctor and related research worker should be made familiar with the ethics of experimentation including the factors which influence its decision making process' (2). Some medical schools, especially in the United States, have developed such teaching already. But in many medical schools and universities discussion on these topics is entirely voluntary, and is organized (if at all) by independent bodies such as the 'London Medical Group'.

Experimentation might be thought to represent a special case, somewhat outside the scope of this paper. But most diagnostic and therapeutic techniques today are so sophisticated and 'scientific', that almost every case becomes, in fact, an experiment in the traditional sense. It may be that the growing reluctance of patients, referred to above, to submit themselves to the rigours of super-scientific medical institutes, represents only one more manifestation of the anti-science trend that is undoubtedly affecting people in the developed countries. In recent years the general public has been opting out of or opting against science to an increasing extent. In view of the very high esteem in which the medical profession has hitherto been held in Western European culture, it would be sad if this trend should start affecting doctor–patient relationships just when medicine is priding itself on becoming more rational and effective than ever before in its history. It would be not only sad, but rather surprising in view of the way in which advances (or 'changes' at any rate) in medical technology have generally been received in the past. Historically, most technical procedures in medicine, however bizarre, have been overvalued by the public, and greeted with enthusiasm, provided only that they were recognized as being directed towards the cure or alleviation of disease. The initial overvaluing of cardiac transplants was absolutely in line with the general tradition. One thinks, for instance, of the remarkable vogue, particularly in the eighteenth and nineteenth centuries, of 'bleeding'. The profession engaged in a veritable orgy of blood-letting for many decades. The instrument employed for the purpose, that 'minute instrument of mighty mischief' as Marshall Hall described the lancet (3, 4, 5) when he urged a more reasonable policy in this matter, was so powerful a symbol of good medical practice that it lent its name to a most distinguished clinical journal. The history of the extravagances of venesection, as practised not merely by the careless or ignorant, but also by men who were both eminent and good thinkers, provides a salutory correction for those who currently overvalue its opposite, namely venepuncture followed by transfusion with a wide range of fluids. A clinical student recently told me that they had been taught that this technique represented 'one of the greatest advances of modern medicine'. In face of such typical hyperbole it is well to remember that not so *very* long ago the same would have been said for venesection, used both prophylactically and therapeutically. Anyone who did not assent to its use in almost all cases was regarded as wholly out of date. Today, the reverse procedure (putting blood and other fluids *into* the blood stream) has become almost routine clinical practice. Now just as one could once have seen the deleterious effects of indiscriminate venesection at autopsy if one had been looking for them, so today, not infrequently, one can see in the post-mortem room (if one cares to look) the results of over-enthusiastic transfusions. Sometimes every soft tissue in the body oozes and drips with excess fluid: fluid administered, perhaps, because a routine laboratory report had suggested a shift in electrolyte balance, or because the patient had had a falling blood pressure. Conscientious clinicians will, of course, say that harm results only from 'bad medicine', and will imply that 'bad medicine' is simply not tolerated in their own wards. Autopsy reports must be the final judge of that kind of assertion, and it has been argued above that special attention should be given to this area of inquiry.

When intravenous fluids are administered (as they often are) in order to correct an electrolyte imbalance reported by the laboratory, a very curious rationale seems to be at work in the mind of the attending clinician. It might be worth looking into its background. It is as though any parameter which appears to be slightly out of line, no matter how fortuitously the 'fact' (and laboratory errors are frequent enough to make any critical mind suspect a single numerical reading) has been discovered, and despite any lack of clinical signs that the patient is actually *ill* because of it, must at all costs be brought back to what is conceived to be a more 'normal' level. The determination to correct what appear to be deviant physical and chemical parameters is a direct consequence of the insistence in modern textbooks on the overriding significance of Cannon's concept of homoeostasis (6). This concept was foreshadowed by Claude Bernard's recognition of the 'constancy of the *milieu intérieur*'. His name does not figure in the bibliographies given by the contributors to the Symposium of 1963, organized by the Society of Experimental Biology, on 'Homoeostasis and Feedback Mechanisms' (7), but it is clear that he adumbrated the concept of homoeostasis while lecturing at the Natural History Museum in Paris in the summer of 1870. In this series of 'Leçons sur les phénomènes de la vie communs aux animaux et aux végétaux' he made one of his best-known aphorisms: 'la fixité du milieu intérieur est la condition de la vie libre, indépendante' (8). That statement embodies a profound insight into the nature of 'free, independent life', which modern understanding (or lack of it) concerning 'la fixité du milieu intérieur' has stood on its head. We should not blame Bernard for those indiscriminate and dangerous attempts to correct deviations from the norm by physical and chemical means, such as are constantly made in hospital wards today: they stem rather from the mechanistic philosophy of biology of Descartes. Claude Bernard would have had little time for the somewhat thoughtless meddling with vital control mechanisms that has resulted, which are sometimes more likely to prevent the body from achieving its 'aim' of free independent life than to assist it in the process. Bernard's attitude towards 'mechanized medicine' is shown in a passage from the second volume of the work (8):

> Quant aux idées de Descartes, elles furent adoptées par un certain nombre de médecins physiologistes et devinrent le fondement d'une doctrine qui jeta un certain éclat, *l'iatromécanique*. Descartes avait posé les premiers principes et appliqué ses idées mécaniques à la structure du corps de l'homme. Ses adeptes étendirent et précisèrent les explications mécaniques des phénomènes vitaux.... *L'iatrochimie* n'est, en quelque sorte, qu'une face de l'iatromécanique. Avant même que la chimie fût constituée, à l'époque où l'on supposait et soupçonnait les phénomènes chimiques plutôt qu'on ne les connaissait, on

avait songé à utiliser ces connaissances rudimentaires pour l'explication des phénomènes vitaux.

It is, to me, somewhat surprising that no English translation has yet been published of this greatest of the works of Claude Bernard, whose earlier *Introduction to the Study of Experimental Medicine* (1865) is well-known and highly regarded. The opportunity to publish in the centenary year of the delivery of the lectures is now gone. A publication timed for the centenary of his death (and of the original publication in French) in 1878, might go far in helping medical technology to contribute more effectively than it currently does to medical services and patient care. Claude Bernard was not only one of the greatest physiologists of all time: he was also a considerable philosopher, who could cut his way through jungles of philosophico-physiological verbiage with the greatest skill. One cannot read him carefully and remain naïve about the attempt to reduce biological phenomena to those of physics and chemistry.

It is sometimes said that new techniques in medical technology (the stock example being the introduction by Jenner of the technique of vaccination) are accepted with as much difficulty and delay as is commonplace with new insights in 'pure science'. Despite all the evident conservatism of human beings, I do not believe that to be so. It seems more likely that opposition to Jenner was based more on emotional repugnance to a hypothesis founded on the transfer of impure material from cows to human beings. But even then the opposition was short-lived, and vaccination rapidly became established as a routine procedure. The success of this technique has in turn given birth, of course, to a whole panoply of preventive techniques (some of doubtful validity) based on the concept of immunity. By and large, man tends uncritically to seize on new medical facilities, always in the hope that somehow they will prevent his being swept down the ever-flowing stream to disease and death. The situation is different in 'pure' science, where opposition to new ideas can be indulged in at a purely rational level, without much emotional involvement—not that that does not happen too, at a personal or individual level. But a technique which claims to alleviate pain and suffering, and even to postpone or abolish death, seems always destined to get an enthusiastic reception. The gullibility not only of the general public, but of scientists and doctors too, over the efficacy of new techniques, whether iatromechanical or iatrochemical (to use Claude Bernard's expressive terms) is profound. Recent examples include not only the extravagant enthusiasm for heart-transplant, but also the banner headlines that greet any report, however flimsy, that suggests a 'breakthrough', say, in cancer control. Mankind is scared of suffering and death. His fear makes him an easy prey to optimism where medical technology is concerned. It is this same enthusiasm, stemming essentially from anxiety, that provides the money for further advances in medical technology, and one is grateful for it, as a practising biological scientist. But is it the need to believe in magical cures (aided and abetted by the advertisement industry) that has made us, for instance, into a society of pill-pushers and pill-swallowers, with a different pill for every complaint? In a context like this, we rapidly come to think of the human frame in a narrowly mechanical way, one that demands the application of mechanical and chemical techniques for every separate, specialized piece of the machinery.

Such gullibility and enthusiasm for a special *technē* was never, perhaps, better illustrated than in the seventeenth century, with the use of 'weapon-salve' (9) as a therapy for the cure of a wound by treating with the instrument that caused it. The mythology involved is at the opposite extreme to our modern, fragmented system of thought. The magical (as we now see it) 'magnetical cure' was interpreted as due to the 'long arm of sympathy' operating in the cosmos, analogous to the similar 'action at a distance' illustrated (against much initial opposition) by the newly discovered Newtonian forces of gravity. Lynn Thorndike dealt somewhat unfairly (10), it seems to me, with one of the main protagonists of the virtue of 'weapon-salve' or 'sympathetic powder', Sir Kenelm Digby. Thorndike accepts without question the vilifications by Evelyn and Stubbes that appear in the *Dictionary of National Biography*, and he too readily dismisses Digby as one of those curious, diplopic alchemical figures of the seventeenth century, with one eye vaguely on science and one firmly fixed on medieval magic and superstition. Joseph Needham, on the other hand, in a more sympathetic study (11), regards Digby as one of the most underestimated figures in the history of seventeenth-century biology where, as he says 'his place is in reality a very high one'. However irrational we may think, today, the whole concept of the weapon-salve to have been, its rationale was argued with great astuteness by its contemporary advocates. The occasional apparent success of the treatment was enough, as always, to promote its use on a wide scale. Can we be so sure, we who in this century have seen the waxing and waning of so many widespread medical fashions, that future generations will not look on us as pityingly as Thorndike looked on some of his characters in his history of magic?

This paper has criticized many of the uses (or, rather, the abuses) of modern medical technology. I should not like it to be thought that I am attacking medical technology as such, or that I am necessarily advocating either a pause in its further development, or a reduction in its use. On the contrary, I would want to welcome every advance in medical technology in the way that Hippocrates would have done, in the way that one welcomes increase in understanding in any area dealing with natural phenomena. What we are most in need of (and so rarely see amongst the clinical experts and specialists in our midst) is a measure of *humility* about our real understanding (as against that 'rudimentary understanding' of which Claude Bernard spoke in the passage quoted above) of that infinitely complex product of the evolutionary process, the living human being. When I consider the sheer power, for both good and harm, that resides in such a simple technical procedure as setting up an intravenous saline drip, I am frightened for the safety of the patient. Perhaps I personally feel this especially because in recent years my major contact with the profession has been through medical students, especially in their early years, before they have developed the cloak of jargon with which to cover the all-too-frequent nakedness of their powers of reasoning. When I watch my students over their years of training, and subsequently in practice, I am not often moved radically to revise my early estimates of their innate intellectual capacities. And I then have genuine fear when I reflect on the enormous powers that they possess with modern sophisticated techniques of iatrophysics and iatrochemistry.

What I would urge, for real improvement of medical services (patient care) by further *understanding* of and advances in medical technology, is the increasing use of modern facilities such as computer programming. I realize that there may be some readers, who have felt sympathetic to the general argument of this chapter, who might experience a sense of shock on reading this last sentence; especially so since the chapter is reaching its end (which is the only part, often, to be read!) and it might be thought that the author is now in the 'opposite camp' of technocrats. I share many of the misgivings of colleagues about the use or abuse of the computer in medicine, particularly in relation to 'medical services' or 'patient care'. What I want to emphasize is that, in itself, a computer is simply an extension of the *technē*. According to Hippocrates, as stated at the beginning of this paper, there is a correspondence between love of *technē* and love of man. Can the computer be absorbed into *philanthropiē*, or must it be regarded as an enemy, where patient care is concerned? Is it just a rather stupid memory-bank that does not help anybody very much? It seems to me that intelligent use of the computer could give medicine the most powerful, and yet most *in-nocent* (in the literal meaning of the word) technique ever discovered. All knowledge, all understanding, involves four stages, all of them requiring the handling of information. They are, in order, information accumulation, filtering (selection), storage, and retrieval. The last stage involves not simply the regurgitation of data previously 'memorized', but the juxtaposition and synthesis (in both space and time) of data culled from various sources, and at various times. This is the essential element in scientific discovery, in 'insight', in the exercise of clinical 'diagnostic flair'. This is the process that the good clinician uses continually, a process of analysis and synthesis, with many feedback loops, both positive and negative. Cyberneticians refer to the process as 'systems analysis', and this concept marks a radical break with the linear, cause–effect paradigm of 'good' natural science which was at the basis of what Bernard called 'l'iatromécanique' and 'l'iatrochimie'. Because of the complexities involved, and the element of uncertainty that continually creeps into the picture with time, any well-programmed 'systems analysis' operates more like an in-depth analysis of an organic or social 'system' than like an analysis of those 'ordinary' pieces of machinery that have been invented since the Industrial Revolution, and that still seem to provide the model for much clinical practice. Because of its speed of operation, and of the fidelity with which it will handle the accurate (or sometimes, unhappily, inaccurate) information with which it has been fed, the computer is able to solve problems of a complexity that would defeat (by sheer exhaustion) its human equivalent, the properly functioning cerebral cortex. We are only, as yet, at the beginning of what has been called the age of *homo gubernator* (cybernetic man). I see the computer as a tool to help us to a much deeper understanding of the nature of man, of man seen in 'biological space-time'. The problem, with the study of the 'infinitely complex' (which is what man is), is that there are so many variables in his make-up that it is literally impossible to judge safely, in advance, the full effects of any single technical procedure on his over-all well-being. It seems to me that we shall begin to cope adequately with some of the complexities involved only when we are humble enough to say 'this problem is bigger than any of us'. We must call on the resources of memory of data-banks, and the ingenious techniques of systems analysis, in order that we should be able once again to look at the patient as a whole human being, rather than looking at him or her as though he were an isolated thyroid gland, a kidney, a blood-marrow dyscrasia, or whatever the reductionist philosophy might suggest in each particular case. Whatever we do or do not do, it is vitally important *primum non nocere*. At this moment in time it looks as if far too many patients *are* being harmed. We shall learn how not to harm them (by sins of either commission or ommission) only by increasing our knowledge and understanding of man as both product and discoverer of the process of biological evolution. Luddite-like protests against machines themselves, or against the abuses perpetrated with their assistance by modern technocrats, are futile. Medical technology *will* continue to increase in complexity. We must ensure the future of medical technology, as of other branches of both science and art, by a much deeper understanding of their powers, and of their place in the evolutionary process itself.

REFERENCES

1. GARRISON, F. H. (1929) *An Introduction to the History of Medicine*, 4th edn (Philadelphia : W. B. Saunders), p. 807.
2. WEBER, H. R. (ed.). (1969). *Experiments with Man: Report of an Ecumenical Consultation* (Geneva : World Council of Churches; New York : Friendship Press), p. 27.
3. HALL, CHARLOTTE (1861). *Memoirs of Marshall Hall* (London : Bentley), p. 51.
4. BRYAN, L. S. (1964), 'Blood-letting in American medicine 1830–92', *Bull. Hist. Med.* 38, 516–29.
5. MARKHAM, W. O. (1866). *Bleeding and Change of Type of Diseases* (Gulstonian Lectures for 1864) (London : Churchill).
6. CANNON, W. B. (1932). *The Wisdom of the Body* (London : Kegan Paul).
7. SOCIETY OF EXPERIMENTAL BIOLOGY (1964). *Symposium on Homoeostasis and Feedback Mechanisms* (Cambridge University Press).
8. BARNARD, C. (1878) *Leçons sur lès phénomènes de la via communs aux animaux et aux vegetaux* (Paris : Baillière et Fils), vol. i, p. 113; vol. ii (1879), p. 434.
9. DEBUS, A. G. (1964). 'Fludd, Gilbert and the weapon-salve', *J. Hist. Med.* 19, 389–417.
10. THORNDIKE, LYNN (1923–58). *History of Magic and Experimental Science*, 8 vols. (New York : Columbia University Press), vol. 7, pp. 498–512.
11. NEEDHAM, JOSEPH (1959). *History of Embryology*, 2nd edn (Cambridge University Press), pp. 121–30.

Discussion

A general discussion of technology in medicine tends to take the form of a dialogue between those who are concerned about its risks and those who are impressed with its value. Since both sides can produce impressive evidence to support their positions, it is essential to seek an accommodation between them.

The injunction that he should do the patient no harm presents the doctor with incomparably greater difficulty today than in the past. Physicians as well as surgeons are now equipped with formidable tools; it is undeniable that many of them are dangerous and that they are sometimes used unnecessarily in investigation and treatment of disease. Valuable remedies often have undesirable side-effects and many examples could be given of mistreatment, sometimes resulting in death. An investigation at Yale showed that among patients cared for in the general medical service, one in five suffered some untoward effect from a diagnostic or therapeutic procedure, and for one in ten the effect was of sufficient severity to prolong the period in hospital. In a large New York hospital, 5 per cent of patients were found to have been admitted because of the consequences of previous medical therapy. Among the reasons for such figures is the use of hazardous methods of investigation and treatment when other safer and less costly procedures are available. Yet another influence is the premature application of research which is incomplete. This occurred in the treatment of coronary artery disease by anticoagulants and is still seen in the use of radiotherapy in treatment of breast cancer when its value has not been established.

These problems, and others, have resulted from the impact of research on medical practice. The success achieved with penicillin and poliomyelitis vaccine has led to a vast investment in medical research and the results are transforming the practice of medicine. But while there is increased knowledge, there is not yet enough knowledge; it is often possible to prolong life when it is threatened by illness without modifying significantly the underlying disease process.

The problems associated with technology have led to doubts about its application to man. Biology, and particularly human biology, is infinitely more complex than physical science. Yet at a time when physicists and chemists are recognizing the complexities of their subject matter, and when they have become aware of their social and ethical responsibilities, doctors are in danger of relying increasingly on a mechanistic approach.

Yet concern about these issues should lead to attempts to solve the problems associated with technology rather than its rejection. It is, after all, to technology that we owe the rising standard of living and the changes in the physical environment that have been largely responsible for improvement in human health. It is to technology that we must look for advance with many of the residual health problems reviewed earlier in this Symposium. Many examples could be cited in which medical technology is already indispensable in the clinical care of patients, and recognition of the associated problems should not make us lose sight of this central fact. Cardiac transplants (which, incidentally, owe less to technology than some other forms of treatment) and the undue attention devoted to them by journalists, have distracted attention from the remarkable advances made with other forms of transplant. Finally, technology in the form of organic chemistry may provide the means of controlling population growth, probably the most significant contribution of any that remains to be made to human health. Moreover some of the risks referred to earlier are due to human errors in the use of the tools rather than to the nature of the tools themselves. Attention should be directed to investigation and, so far as possible, elimination of those errors.

Notable progress has already been made in this direction. In Britain the Department of Health and Social Security conducts an inquiry into the reasons for every maternal death and there have been similar investigations of perinatal mortality. Anaesthetists in many areas attempt to discover the cause of every death by anaesthesia. Most hospitals in England have ethical committees which have to approve new methods of investigation or treatment before they are applied generally to patients. Attempts are also being made to eliminate prescribing errors by epidemiological methods including, in some cases, the use of computers.

The problems associated with the application of computers illustrate some of the difficulties confronting technology in medicine. This useful tool is probably indispensable for many purposes, for example the discovery and elimination of errors in prescribing and laboratory analysis, as well as for management techniques analogous to those already used widely in business. But it is very doubtful whether computers will transform the practice of medicine by influencing significantly clinical decisions on the diagnosis and treatment of disease; and certainly it cannot replace the general physician, who alone can ensure that his patients get the advantages of technology while being protected so far as is possible from its concomitant risks.

7

ON MEASURING ECONOMIC BENEFITS OF HEALTH PROGRAMMES

RASHI FEIN

On measuring economic benefits of health programmes

1. EARLY HISTORY

> When the sentimentalist and the moralist fails, he will have as a last resource to call in the aid of the economist, who has in some instances proved the power of his art to draw iron tears from the cheeks of a city Plutus (1).

Economic data and analysis have long been used in efforts to influence programme and expenditure decisions in the public sector. Those who have favoured particular policies have sought allies and supporting arguments for their positions. Particularly appealing have been the arguments that were cast in economic terms, and this has, perhaps, been especially the case in areas involving programmes with clear, visible, and direct impact on people. This appeal would appear to have been based on two factors. The general attractiveness of economic arguments has, at least in part, derived from the belief that economics is value-free, neutral, and objective. Thus, economic arguments relying on the hard criteria of the market, on 'profit' and on 'loss', carried a special weight (a weight that was, perhaps, increased by the fact that economists use data, jargon, and methodology that are somewhat mysterious to the uninitiated). The specific attractiveness of economic arguments in social areas (for example in the case of programmes that deal directly with people) is increased by the fact that these fields generally lack rigorous monetary guidelines for decision-making. In Chadwick's terms, these are the areas favoured by 'the sentimentalist and moralist'.

Therefore, to find that economic criteria were not at variance with humanitarian considerations seemed to be especially useful. Chadwick was correct when he suggested that the economist could prove a useful ally.

The power of the economic argument that the proponents of social programmes found useful was not derived from the literary quality with which the arguments were offered, or from the elegance of the economist's prose. Nor, as will become clear, did it result from the fact that the analytical methodology was so refined and the data so exact that disagreement with the conclusions was impossible. Rather it was because the economic argument embodied an appealing pattern of thought and a way of looking at a problem: the economic rationale for various social programmes was presented in investment terms. Ill-health, ignorance, disability, and death caused by war were costly to an economy. Investment in medical care, public health, education, and in the pursuit of peace, brought significant economic rewards in increasing the value of human capital. Such investment concepts were looked upon with favour at a time when economic progress was seen as deriving from capital growth brought about by investment.

Thus, the early literature of economics as well as articles in applied areas of public policy, contains references to the economic value of an education, of acquired skills, of better health, and to the economic costs and gains of war, emigration, and immigration. These subjects were examined at irregular intervals by persons concerned with practical policy matters. Unfortunately none of these contributions developed a general theory and methodology concerning the economic value of a human being. They were not integrated into the main body of the economic literature, remaining on, if not beyond, the fringe. Furthermore, because they were derived from a specific interest in a particular applied problem, there was little attempt to generalize or to show the usefulness of the approach to other problems. Those writing on the economic value of an immigrant seemed unaware that a similar type of problem was examined by persons concerned with the economic value of an education;

those writing on the economic loss suffered through emigration seemed unaware that other scholars were concerned with the economic loss caused by disease or by casualties in war.

This situation, I might note, makes the examination of early references to human capital a fascinating but time-consuming task. Some years ago, in undertaking just such an examination, I found that in order to locate useful examples of the quantitative application of the concept of human capital, one had to consider the various fields in which such a concept might be used and then search for articles, bibliographies, and references in these applied fields. General indexes were hardly useful since they contained no classification heading called human resources or human capital. Even titles of articles could be, and were, misleading.

Perhaps the first estimates of the money value of a person were offered by Sir William Petty writing in the latter decades of the seventeenth century. At various times Petty offered estimates of the value of a person residing in England. These estimates ranged between £60 and £90. In his *Political Arithmetick*, for example, Petty calculates the value by deriving the productive contributions of labour (£26 million), multiplying by 20 ('The Mass of Mankind being worth Twenty Years purchase . . .') and by dividing by 6 million (the population of England). Thus '. . . makes about £80. Sterling, to be valued of each Head of Man Woman and Child . . .: from whence we may learn to compute the loss we have sustained by the Plague, by the Slaughter of Men in War, and by the sending them abroad into the Service of Foreign Princes' (2). Petty then used estimates of the value of human capital to derive a number of policy implications. He asked: 'From whence it follows, that 100,000 persons dying of the Plague, above the ordinary number is near 7 Millions loss to the Kingdom [this was based upon an estimate that each person was worth £69]; and consequently how well might £70,000 have been bestowed in preventing this Centuple loss?' (3). In another work he asked: 'The value of 140^{m} people at £90. per head is 12 millions 600^{m} pounds; soe as the Question seems to be what sum of money, and Meanes ought to be prudently ventured for the probable cutting off 3 fifths of this Calamity' (4). In Petty's plan, dated 7 October 1667, 'Of Lesening ye Plagues of London', he attempted to provide an answer to the question. He estimated that, given the value of an individual and the cost of transporting people outside of London and caring for them for three months, thus increasing the probability of survival, every pound expended would yield a return of £84 (5). Here, then, was an economic argument, cast in monetary terms, in favour of a course of action to prevent deaths and thus to increase the value of the nation's human resources.

Petty also used the concept of human capital in advocating lying-in hospitals for illegitimate children. He calculated that the cost of thirty days in child-bed would only be 30*s*. Since the value of mankind was some £70 'a new born Child, bread up to fair and hard work for 25 yeares, will be very well worth 3 times 30 Shillings, as may be seen in the price of Negros Children in the American plantations' (4). It is not without interest to note that Petty advocated lying-in hospitals in order to increase the population. Perhaps, however, to insure that the government receive a direct return on its investment, he also advocated that the child should be the servant of government for twenty-five years. Today, with the growth of income taxation, the argument is often made in terms of the direct returns to government resulting from the increase in tax revenue.

Some twenty-one years earlier, in 1676, in a lecture on anatomy, Petty noted that the state should intervene to assure better medicine. The value of better medicine, he felt, was that it could save 200,000 subjects a year. Even valued at only £20, the lowest price of slaves, this was a large sum and better medicine, therefore represented a sensible state expenditure. 'Wherefore it is not in the Interest of the State to leave Phisitians and Patients (as now) to their own shifts' (6). Almost three hundred years later, the same arguments are presented (though the data are more refined) to advocate similar policies.

It is also of interest to note that not only was Petty the precurser of present discussions of investment in health activities, but he also presented arguments analogous to those used today in discussions concerning migration and economic development policies. Petty argued that an individual in England was worth £90, but that in Ireland only £70. This differential value led to the conclusion that transplantation would be economically wise (4).

Over a century passes before the economic value of man concept reappears again in a major way in the literature. Edwin Chadwick, in his *Sanitary Report* for 1842, estimated that the loss due to excessive sickness and premature disability and death, including the loss of productive power equalled £14 million (7). In 1844 he argued that bad sanitation increased the proportion of dependent hands to workers and that sanitation could be viewed 'as an economical question of production' (8). He also suggested that it could be shown 'how much, by expenditure in well-executed measures, directed by engineering science, they may gain in the reduction of existing pecuniary burdens alone, that are entailed by an excessive mortality' (10). Chadwick, of course, was particularly interested in sanitation, and a number of his many articles contain references to the economic value of sanitation and to the costs that society bears in '. . . excessive sickness, excessive death-rates and funerals, and premature disablement and lost labour . . .' due to poor sanitation (9).

In 1862, Chadwick argued, '. . . as the artist for his purpose views the human being as a subject for the cultivation of the beautiful—as the physiologist for the cultivation of his art views him solely as a material organism, so the economist for the advancement of his science may well treat the human being simply as an investment of capital, in productive force' (1). He then presented detailed estimates of the value of a person based on the cost of rearing a child, taking account of the factor of death before becoming productive (at age 11!) and the number of productive years. He used these estimates to derive the costs associated with poor housing and sanitation, and offered additional comments related to the value of human capital. Suggesting that economists should strive to unite personal and pecuniary motives, he defended education on economic grounds and, in words which remain applicable today, argued: '. . . it is well to subscribe to reformatories as to hospitals for the treatment of the sick, but giving exclusive attention to them is like giving exclusive attention to the foundation and maintenance of hospitals for the alleviation of marsh and foul air diseases, without regard to the drainage of the marshes, or to the removal of the sources of the foul air whence the diseases arise' (1).

Lemuel Shattuck in the *Report of a General Plan for the Promotion of Public and Personal Health*, presented in 1850, also viewed public health measures from an economic perspective. In arguing for preventive sanitary measures to lessen epidemics, he wrote: 'In this case economy is on the side of humanity, and the most expensive of all things is—to do nothing' (10). The expenses and losses caused by the neglect of sanitary measures included 'A loss sustained by the state, in consequence of the diminished physical power and general liability to disease' (10). Shattuck estimated that the failure of the State of Massachusetts to adopt an efficient sanitary system resulted in 6,000 unnecessary deaths and that the average individual might have been productive for an additional eighteen years. Thus, society lost 108,000 years of labour at $50 per year, equalling $5·4 million. When this was added to the lost labour of the sick, the cost of sickness and of supporting widows and orphans, Shattuck estimated that the cost to the state was $7·5 million. Interestingly, he felt that this cost could be eliminated by an expenditure of only $3,000 (largely in planning and, what we would call today 'technical assistance') (10). Shattuck thus argued:

According to the estimate above presented, the State suffers, from its imperfect sanitary condition, an unnecessary annual loss of more than 7½ millions of dollars! and this arises, partly at least, from the non-adoption of a measure which will cost but about $3,000. If saved, it would add that amount to the wealth of the State, besides the indefinite amount of increased happiness which would accompany it. Should any one consider this an extravagant estimate, let him reduce it to 3 millions, more than one half, and then the relation of expenditure to the savings, or to the income, will be as *one dollar* to *one thousand dollars*! And even if nine tenths of this latter sum be deducted, it will be like paying out *one* dollar, and receiving back again *ten*, as the return profit! What more wise expenditure of money can be desired? (10).

In the latter half of the nineteenth century others were writing in much the same vein as Chadwick and applying the same concepts to a number of different fields. They would have accepted the statement by the Revd J. E. Thorold Rogers: 'It seems to me wholly un-philosophical to ignore capital in the person of a labourer, and to recognize it in a machine' (11). One writer, however, stands out above all others because of the method by which he calculated what he termed the 'money value of a man' and because he applied the concept to general taxation problems as well as to social programmes. William Farr, in a paper presented in 1853 discussing income and property taxes, used a method that is surprisingly close to the methods used today since he did not base values on the costs of rearing the child (producing the machine) but rather on the wages that will be earned, on the future income stream (12). In his volume *Vital Statistics*, Farr stated:

> Life has a pecuniary value. In its production and education a certain amount of capital is sunk for a longer or shorter time, and that capital, with its interest, as a general rule, reappears in the wages of the labourer, the pay of the officer, and the income of the professional man. At first it is all expenditure, and a certain necessary expenditure goes on to the end to keep life in being, even when its economic results are negative (13).

The sum of future earnings and the cost of future maintenance determines the value. Thus Farr estimates the following values for a Norfolk agricultural labourer: at birth £5; age 5, £56; age 10, £117; age 15, £192; age 20, £234; age 25, £246; age 30, £241 declining to £138 at age 55, and £1 at age 70, following which the values become negative (maintenance exceeds income) and, thus, at age 80 the value is −£41. Farr uses these data to justify particular concern with those events that destroy lives at their prime—'fever, consumption, cholera, violence in all its forms, and childbirth' (13).

The estimates provided by Farr in his *Vital Statistics* that a human life was worth $770 a head were used by Gary Calkins in estimating that sanitation saved 856,804 lives with a value of $650 million from 1880 to 1890. This saving, he noted, exceeded the cost of sanitary improvements between 1875 and 1890, since the latter totalled $583·5 million (14).

If Petty was the first to examine the concept of human capital and Chadwick the first to present detailed estimates and apply these quite carefully and extensively to justify various public expenditures, Farr deserves recognition as the first to analyse value in terms of future income streams and to do this in relation to the general question of taxation rather than in a specific context of health (or other) expenditures.

In the period 1870–1920, the concept of human capital continued to be applied in a number of specific areas. The economic value of man entered into discussions on the cost of war (perhaps with the hope that war would be eliminated if it were recognized that when the loss in human capital was included in the 'profit and loss statement' even the victor could be found to have made a poor investment). Detailed studies on the cost of the Franco-Prussian War of 1870 were undertaken (chiefly by Sir Robert Giffen). Additional studies on the South African War and the First World War included estimates of the production foregone during the war (because men were in the armed forces) as well as losses due to deaths and injuries (15–18).

A second group of economists applied the concept of human capital to problems of emigration and immigration. British writers tended to focus on the loss that Britain was suffering because of emigration. Migration, it was felt, represented the loss of a capital asset (though the value of the asset was not always measured in terms of future income, but on occasion in terms of the cost of 'creating' the asset; for example, the cost of upbringing and education). Archibald Hamilton, writing in 1877, noted that the value of an immigrant to the community has been estimated in the United States at £166. 13*s*. 4*d*. and 'they have been computed to be worth £200 in New Zealand' (11). In response, Dr Guy suggested that the value of an immigrant was £400 'and when it was remembered that an emigrant . . . married and became the father of children who . . . had families, it was difficult to say what the true value of an emigrant was' (20). There was general agreement, however, that the value of an immigrant depended upon the demand for labour in the place to which he emigrated. Thus Farr noted that the ex-Prime Minister of New Zealand, Sir Julius Vogel, had done 'An admirable work . . . to remove some of the agricultural labourers from a place where they were worth very little, to a place where they were worth a great deal' (20).

A third area of economic inquiry that utilized a capital concept of man dealt with health and with the costs associated with specific diseases. Among the diseases studied were tuberculosis and typhoid fever (21–2). These studies did not break new methodological ground, nor did they lead the general economist to a greater interest in the field of health. Just as the profession neglected the field of human resources in general, so too, it neglected the area of health.

It is not clear why there was relatively little discussion of the economic value of human resources, except by scholars interested in applied specific problem areas. Economists, after all, have long referred to land, labour, and capital inputs and resources. They have devoted considerable analysis to the consequences derived from the observed fact that land is not homogeneous and from the observation that capital equipment differs in its productivity. Yet, to a considerable extent, much of economics has been written as if labour were all the same. Even when cognizance was taken of the obvious and observable differences in labour quality, there seemed to be little concern with analysis of the factors that brought about these differences, almost as if it were felt that the factors could not be controlled or were not amenable to change. It is significant, perhaps, that to the extent that human capital was considered (even by those in applied areas), greatest attention was paid to problems of mortality, total incapacity, or migration—issues involving the addition or subtraction of total productivity rather than an increase in productivity resulting from the individual's becoming more effective in his work.

We can only speculate why human capital was largely ignored by the main body of economics. In part it may be due to the fact that during the period of rapid economic growth (the period of rapid industrial growth and the period when economics was developing as an organized discipline), striking and rapid changes were taking place in the amount of capital equipment available to the society and at the disposal of the worker. The capital/labour ratio was increasing. It is, therefore, to be expected that capital equipment occupied the centre of the stage and was the chief focus of interest. Higher standards of living were seen as the result of the process of industrialization. Industrialization, in turn, was seen as the consequence (synonomous with) investment in addition to the stock of capital equipment. Changes in the quality of human resources were not as obvious, certainly not as easy to measure or as dramatic, not as apparently the result of deliberate policies. Thus, they were given small parts in the chorus along with other actors called custom, organization, entrepreneurship, and so forth.

Secondly, capital and differences in capital could easily be measured in economic terms. Capital is traded in the market and no conversion to economic or monetary terms is required. The common denominator that expresses the value of capital equipment is there for all to see. One-time investments in capital yield future income streams. Labour, however, is not bought and sold. Only labour services are. In general (with exceptions in discussions of insurance), one did not think in terms of income streams when discussing labour.

Thirdly, labour plays a dual role in the economic system: as input and as final consumer. Many of the things that increase the value and contribution of the worker as input (things that could be termed investments) are considered as part of consumption. They involve expenditures on goods and services that, in many cases, would be purchased even if they did nothing to improve the skill levels and productivity of the working force. Thus, the costs of recreation are classified as consumption expenditures even if they might be considered as part of the necessary costs required to maintain productivity. So, too, with health expenditures and with education expenditures. Surely people want health and education, and would purchase some of these two commodities, even in the absence of any impact on productivity and earning power? Surely, however, health and education do have such impacts and are not, therefore, entirely consumption expenditures? Some portion can be viewed (and in recent years this has been the case) as investment.

Fourth, the early orientation of economics failed to take account of the importance of 'externalities'. Expenditures on health and education that increased the productivity of the worker were viewed as private matters since they increased the individual's income. It was not fully appreciated that all of us are the beneficiaries when some of us are more productive. Nor was it recognized that certain expenditures might make sound economic sense for society as a whole even though they did not do so for the individual. If externalities are ignored much of the rationale for public intervention disappears—much, but not all—and with a weaker rationale there was a lesser interest in such, clearly, private matters.

Fifth, economists, as others, failed to examine some expenditures as investments and failed to view human capital as capital, at least in part because the terminology was felt repellent when applied to man. Man is not a machine. How then could one use such terms as 'human capital' or 'investment in human beings'. The notion of man as something that can be assigned some dollar value reminds one of slavery. It seems to violate the concept of the sacredness of life. The notion is rejected as repugnant. Even when the ideas are explored and man is assigned an economic value, writers often felt it necessary to make disclaimers that man is much more than a robot merely embodying some set of skills. The fact that the writer felt that he might be misunderstood in the absence of such disclaimers is in itself significant.

In recent years, however, there has been a significant change in the place that human resources occupy in the literature of economics. The 1950s saw rekindled interest in health economics and the economics of education. This was built upon in the decade of the 1960s as economists turned their attention to a variety of issues relating to investment in human capital. No longer were these considered fringe areas. Today there is a field known as the economics of human resources. There are economists, courses, workshops, seminars, conferences, and a journal —perhaps the final evidence that a field exists—devoted to this area of inquiry. In little more than a decade the situation has changed from the case where individuals, who had not yet succeeded in defining a field or having it accepted by their professional colleagues, were working in relative isolation on problems that today would be defined as part of the 'economics of human resources'. In the course of this change, there has been an altered orientation to the questions that have been studied. It is to this altered orientation, particularly as it applies to questions in the health areas, that we now turn.

2. RECENT DEVELOPMENTS

We recall that many of the early contributions already referred to were designed to promote specific policies by demonstrating that funds expended for various social programmes would bring economic returns. Economists or their analytical techniques were called upon 'when the sentimentalist and the moralist' needed additional support. In this heavily investment-oriented approach one discovers little reference to programmes that do not yield a high return. Nor do we find suggestions that expenditures for certain activities should be cut. This may be because economists chose not to address problems that might yield 'negative' answers, because they chose not to publish 'negative' results, or because there are few, if any, general social programmes that have very low yields. While there may have been an element of the first two reasons—most of the articles, after all, were written by persons actively working in and dedicated to action in the particular applied field—the last reason is, perhaps, of even greater importance. The absence of low rates of return is particularly true if the analysis is cast in general and broad dimension rather than as an examination of a specific programme, designed to accomplish a narrow and specific purpose in which the outcome can be measured. What was being evaluated was whether better health or more education had a substantial payoff, not whether this particular educational technique raised reading levels to a degree commensurate with the resources required to implement the technique or whether a particular health programme in a particular location and designed to help a particular population group had a substantial payoff. Most of the literature spoke of health in general, education in general. Most of the literature did not describe the particular programme that would be designed to alter the existing situation and surely did not examine the likelihood that the programme would accomplish its goals. The analysis was based on 'average' data for large population groups and did not concern itself with whether or not the population groups to be served by the expenditures which were being advocated would, in fact, exhibit an average response to the new programme. Given the broad nature of the questions being addressed, it is not surprising that the returns were found to be high.

To be sure, part of the reason that one would expect to find high rates of return also relates to the methodology that was used to calculate the yields (the absence of discounting, for example). This, however, is not the critical element for even today when a more refined methodology (much of which works to lower the calculated rate of return) is utilized, rates remain high when one speaks of education in general (as contrasted with a particular programme for particular students). Similarly, with health.

Even during the 1950s, the decade in which the revival of interest in the economics of human resources began, elements of the older tradition were maintained. Much of the new work undertaken, related to the economic rates of return to various levels of education and the economic costs of various diseases—not to the rate of return to specific education or health programmes. The analysis did, of course, demonstrate that education had a high yield and that disease was costly. It did not ask, however, what specific programmes could—in the real world—lower the incidence of disease and by how much. It did not ask what the rates of return would be for those programmes.

Similarly, it did not ask how learning could be increased and what the returns to new educational programmes were likely to be. Yet, even the work that was done, limited as it was, was extremely important both in introducing economists to various applied fields in the social programme areas and in introducing an economic dimension to the discussion of these kinds of activities.

The reasons for the revival of interest in the economics of health and education in the 1950s are many. Concern about rapidly increasing budgets for education (and to a smaller degree for health) led to attempts to 'justify' those budgets by examination of the economic benefits of education and health activities. Concern about underdeveloped economies brought us face to face with the question of skills and productivity, with the costs to production that result from lack of adequate education and health. It was clear that plant, equipment, roads, and electric power were not enough to insure development, and that quality of the labour force also made a difference. In the United States, concern about Soviet scientific advances and the growth in Soviet Gross National Product led to attempts to put empirical content into the statements that a nation's richest resource was its skilled manpower and that its wealth included its stock of engineers and scientists. Attempts to examine problems of economic growth in developed economies led to intensive examination of the sources of growth. United States Gross National Product, it is clear, has grown more rapidly than can be accounted for by increases in land, labour, and capital. There have, therefore, been attempts to provide more precise measurements and explanations of the part not accounted for, the residual element in growth. While primary emphasis has often been given to research and technology, a spill-over effect has directed considerable attention to capital invested in men. Finally, economists have directed more and more attention not only to income differences between nations but also to differences between groups in the same nation, to the reasons for these differences and to socio-economic policies that might narrow the differences. In the United States, the economic problems of Negroes has been an important focus of interest for economists (and others), and many have attributed much of the income part of the problem to the underinvestment in education and health for this part of our population.

During the 1960s, however, the nature of much of the empirical effort in the economics of health (and of education) began to change. Increasingly, many felt that the work of economists on rates of return was interesting and illuminating, but not very helpful in guiding public policy and in choosing between public programmes. High rates of return are encouraging to the practitioner in a given field and they make for fine banquet address material, but they do not answer two questions that government budgeteers raise: (1) are the specific programmes for which support is sought 'good' investments, i.e., what are the rates of return for the various proposals that come before the decision-maker; (2) which particular programmes should be favoured over other programmes, i.e., how does the rate of return for each programme compare with rates of return for alternatives? In the government sector these are the kinds of questions that are asked and, particularly, in the mid 1960s, the kinds of questions that United States government departments began asking of economists.

It should be remembered that there was a flavour, a 'climate of opinion' in the early 1960s. Ideology was 'dead', and the problems were, to a considerable measure, viewed as technical ones which required 'technical' solutions. The analyst was not only necessary but sufficient. Those were the days of 'the whizz kids' in the Pentagon, those were the days when it was felt that hard intellectual effort, the power of logic, and rationality would provide the answers to the society. In such an atmosphere, the importance of economists in government grew considerably. Thus, economists were among those asking (and answering) the questions of allocation of budget resources.

The issue confronting the budget officer and other decision-makers, after all, is not whether there is or is not (which in terms of the analysis often means 'has or has not been') a high rate of return (an economic payoff) to health activities in general. Government budgets do not allocate funds to health in general but to specific programmes and activities. The question, therefore, is and should be how specific programmes and activities measure up and how they will do *in the future* since the future may differ from the past (if only because the population groups to be served may become successively harder to reach). This is true whether one is conducting an economic analysis or any other type of evaluative effort. Furthermore, the decision-maker does not have free resources. He is subject to a budget constraint. He must *choose* between a large number of alternative programmes. It is, therefore, necessary to compare the likely gains and costs of the various possible courses of action that are open to him. He needs to ask how a particular programme compares with other programmes, how an *incremental* expenditure in one area compares with others.

Thus, in the mid 1960s we witnessed a conscious attempt to utilize the economist's tools in behalf of the decision-maker. Economists, called upon to examine specific programmes, had to shift their attention from the aggregative and macro aspects to the micro level. They were asked to compare programmes and rank them in terms of the relationship between costs and benefits. These economists (and the data for analysis) were most often found in government rather than outside. They were at work for and at the behest of the decision-maker himself, not for persons in an applied area who were trying to influence the decisions in their favour.

It can be noted that the intervention of economists in the process was not without difficulties. There was some controversy whether the analytical effort could best proceed at the highest level, say in the Bureau of the Budget (i.e., the President's staff), in the office of the Secretary of a Department, or in the individual operating agencies. The problem of where to carry forward such work to insure that the analyst has access to data and to the experience of persons intimately acquainted with programme operations and yet does not become a special pleader for the operating agency is important. Though we shall not discuss this at further length, we must note that success or failure in analysis and in influencing the decision-making process may hinge on the locational decision.

We speak of the economist's role in helping conduct *ex-ante* analysis of the consequences of decisions. This attempt often involved the application of quantitative methods to the analysis of the various alternatives open to the decision-maker. If it is granted that the essential characteristic of decision-making is that of choice as between alternatives (including, of course, the option of postponing the decision), then the process of choice involves some kind of a comparison of the likely gains and the likely costs of the various courses of action or inaction. This pattern of thought—though not necessarily in quantitative terms—is applicable to all facets of rational decision-making. Certainly it existed before 1965. What was new was the attempted quantification of costs and benefits, the attention to economic benefits, the involvement of economists, and the attempt to compare programmes in an explicit way. It should be clear, however, that gains and costs need not be limited to or expressed in monetary terms. They must include any number of other considerations which are relevant to the problem or decision at hand: gains or costs in prestige, political fortune, satisfaction, goodwill, effort, energy, and so forth. What is important is that in the evaluation, the comparisons be made explicit. It is also helpful if they be made in units which are commensurable.[1]

That economists were heavily involved thus does not mean that the only benefits that were or need to be considered are economic benefits, though, of course, there is the danger that a particular profession may tend to overlook the importance of things that lie outside its area of professional competence. Economists were involved for many reasons. They had developed a reputation in subjecting public decisions (particularly

1. When the argument is cast in its broadest and most general terms it loses some of its operational significance since it can presumably be argued that when comparisons are not made (and decisions are arrived at on bases that, to some, may appear irrational) that the individual making the decision felt that the benefits of undertaking more refined comparisons and of reaching decisions in a more deliberate and explicit manner were outweighed by the costs involved.

in the areas of water resources and defence) to analysis and in forcing the consideration of alternatives. They were used to empirical methods and to the pattern of thought that explicitly attempts to compare benefits and costs. They were conversant with the language of the men who prepare budgets. Finally, they were viewed as 'objective', i.e., not special pleaders for a particular programme or area.

Perhaps most important, economists had been most concerned with economic growth policies and with measures to increase the rate of growth. Many of the programmes that were to be analysed were examined from the perspective of growth. Furthermore, economists were concerned with the constraint of limited resources and the necessity for choice. The analysis was to involve the comparison of alternatives.

I do not propose to examine the details of the effort begun in the 1960s to bring the new type of analysis to bear on the governmental policy decision-making process. This is not the place to review that history. To do so would require that we move well beyond the area of our specific interests since the analytical effort was tied in with a number of other new activities in the planning and budgeting process, all of them designed collectively to make for better decisions and for wider range of choice. Our purposes are better served by examination of some of the conceptual difficulties that are involved in the effort to assess costs and benefits of programmes for people, particularly programmes which are viewed as human investment programmes. Let us, therefore, examine some of the issues that arise and that are involved in the quantitative analysis of benefits and costs.

3. CONCEPTUAL ISSUES

Basic to all considerations of programmes is the need to specify the objectives of the programme in question and to develop techniques and reporting systems that enable one to assess the degree to which the objectives are being met. It is clear that these are first and important steps. It is also clear that, in many cases, these steps entail great difficulty. The difficulties arise in part because the final objectives of many government programmes are to produce outputs which, at least at the present time, cannot be measured directly. The difficulties also arise because, often, we know relatively little about the production process whereby these final outputs are created. I do not ignore the difficulties involved in creating data and reporting systems to measure the achievement of limited and well-defined goals (e.g., reduction in incidence of a particular disease). In no small measure our relative ignorance about many health matters relates to the fact that our data systems are underdeveloped and —in terms of funds and personnel—undernourished. Far too often we simply do not have the data we need for analytical purposes. These difficulties, however, are surmountable, and better reporting and data systems can be created. I refer instead to the even greater problems associated with the measurement of outputs which are amorphous in concept, outputs such as 'higher levels of health' and which are contributed to by many factors (e.g., housing, income, nutrition, environment, medical care of all kinds), factors whose relative contribution may differ for different persons and whose relative contribution is largely unknown.

The difficulty of measuring the achievement of goals which lie on a continuum is apparent. We do not do as well in measuring pain, concern, or functional ability, as we do in measuring states which are discontinuous, such as life and death. Two consequences arise as a result of the problem of measurement and of understanding how various states of health are or can be produced. First, our lack of understanding of the production process and our inability to measure outputs leads programme administrators to define their goals in resource input terms: the goal is more hospital beds, more physicians, more patient visits, more examinations, more research, above all more money. It is an article of faith that good things are accomplished by more resources and that things will be even better if even more resources are utilized. This may indeed be the case, but it is not the issue for the question must be, 'how much better'. It is analogous to saying that a health programme is effective because it produces a positive change. The argument that we present says that that is not a sufficient guideline to the policy-maker since he must choose between different programmes and, therefore, must be concerned with levels of effectiveness. His concern cannot be with whether a form of treatment or a government programme is likely to do some good, but rather with the amount of good accomplished per unit of resource input. He cannot be satisfied with a goal of more inputs, unless he understands how inputs relate to outputs, in which case he might as well speak in output terms.

There exists a second important consequence of our difficulty in measuring outputs. This arises most often in the development of new programme alternatives. The pressure to quantify, to measure, to be able to assess whether the goal is being achieved and in what degree, creates a bias in favour of developing those programmes that have output goals that can be measured, where data can be gathered, where the achievement of limited (but specified) goals can be documented. These, however, are not necessarily the most desirable, needed, or highest yield programmes. They may be, but they need not be.

The problem of measurement of output is a real one and the consequences are real as well. There is no reason, however, to be totally pessimistic about their solution. First, we must recognize that except for the bias in selection of programmes (a bias which I believe can be guarded against) these problems leave us no worse off than we are in the absence of the evaluation effort. It is not the attempt to calculate cost-benefit ratios that leaves us at sea, that makes us ignorant of production functions and forces us to speak of inputs rather than of outputs. These problems are with us all the time. Indeed the cost-benefit analysis leads to a greater level of understanding of the deficiencies in our measurement techniques, of the vagueness of some of our goals. It does not make us ignorant but makes us aware of our ignorance. It forces us to question the 'conventional wisdom'—a discreet phrase that often really means well-accepted, but not fully documented, professional judgements. In the long run—and because of the recognition of the inadequate state of our knowledge—many of the problems will be partially solved. Some of them, I believe, are not fully solvable since they involve interpersonal comparisons and changing standards of need and adequacy, and thus changing measurements of the benefits derived from various programmes. In the short run (and the short run may be a very long time indeed), we will be forced to find proxy measures for the outputs that are our ultimate interests. Thus, even if we are unable to develop a satisfactory index of health, there would be agreement that the absence of illness—while not a fully satisfactory measure of health—might serve as one of a number of proxy measures. It is necessary, of course, to be careful not to subvert the real aims of a programme by adjusting it to serve the proxy measure—a programme designed to improve the health of children with the consequence that they have fewer days of absence from school (the proxy measure) is different from a programme that focuses so heavily on the proxy that its attempt to achieve success leads sick children to be sent to school, perhaps contributing to even more illness. The danger that new (and measurable) aims are substituted for the real ones can, however, be guarded against.

Let us assume that, alert to the difficulties and biases and the dangers that they entail, the goals of the programmes have been specified and measures of the outputs have been developed. The difficulties are not yet over. Since the interest lies in the comparison of programmes, there develops a need to find a common denominator for the different outputs, a way of translating different things into a common unit of measure, a way, for example, of comparing the value of a life saved with a case of blindness prevented, of the life of a 10-year-old with the life of a 50-year-old, and so forth.

As has already been pointed out, these kinds of questions (e.g., the value of human life) are often found to be distasteful. None the less, whether formulated explicitly or implicitly, they are being asked—and are being answered—all the time. Often, however, because they are not formulated explicitly, one may find that governments pursue expenditure policies that imply that some lives are worth much more than others (e.g., aeroplane passengers as contrasted with coalminers). Thus, distasteful as it may be to articulate these types of questions, it is better that we do so than that we reach policy decisions without being explicitly aware of their value implications.

The search for a common unit of measurement is, however, fraught with danger. We are unable to measure units of satisfaction or of happiness generated by various government activities. Nor are we able to compare *A*'s satisfaction with *B*'s. None the less, the climate of opinion places a premium on measurement. Since the evaluation of alternative programmes is carried forward by economists who are responding to budget and treasury officials, themselves sensitive to data that are presented in financial terms, and since the evaluation of programmes is being undertaken in an atmosphere that is investment and economic growth-oriented (while in the United States this atmosphere may be changing—one hopes that is the case—cost-benefit and programme analysis is still too young to have outgrown its early and very recent history), the common denominator that is most often sought is a monetary unit and the benefits most often measured are monetary ones. The fact that the monetary benefits are measured does not imply that economists are less concerned about other benefits than are historians, philosophers, or the general public. It simply means that economists (as others) tend to measure that which is measurable and tend first to address their attention to those things that they are familiar with: dollar costs and dollar benefits. Thus, as with the writings of economists and others in an earlier period, benefits are often translated into dollars (more correctly, the benefits that are measured are those that can be cast in dollar terms). This is the case even though it is total benefits of all kinds that we are interested in. Monetary benefits are—at best—only a proxy for total benefits. They are only part (perhaps only a small part) of all benefits and do not represent a stable or constant fraction of all benefits. The problems that may, therefore, arise are many.

In measuring the economic benefits of programmes it has become traditional to assess the increase in earning power of the individual that results from the improved health brought about by the programme under review. The increase in earning power is a measure of the gain to the economy since the contribution to production is measured by wages and salary income. This is not different from the evaluation made by those whose writings we examined above. It will be recalled that in those writings the value of a human being was assessed in different ways at different times: sometimes in terms of the cost of rearing (of producing the 'machine') but later—and as is still done today—in terms of future earnings, a measure of expected future productive contribution. Using this measure entails some decisions about conceptual problems: what value should be placed on productive contribution and work effort that does not receive monetary rewards through the market system, a problem not confined to but often found in the case of women; what adjustments, if any, should be made to the gross earnings figure to take account of the individual's consumption; should adjustment be made for the additional investments that the individual or that society might make in the future in order to increase the individual's skills and his productive contribution and his earning power; what account should be taken of unemployment at the national level and at the regional level (what assumptions are reasonable as regards mobility and migration); should the future earnings figures be adjusted when there is evidence that because of market imperfections the individual is being rewarded at too low a rate?[1] These and numerous other issues arise and require a measure of agreement. Important as these issues are, we can only note them. Our discussion moves on to two matters that, it seems to me, are particularly troublesome.

The first issue, not unlike some of the difficulties that we have discussed earlier, relates to the problems and biases that may

1. Market imperfections arise in many areas. As early as 1861, it was suggested that '. . . the value of compulsory servitude in the Army . . . (should include) . . . the value between the market price of labour and the price paid for it by government . . .' (23). This issue has, once again, arisen in the debates in the United States concerning the comparison of the cost of a volunteer and of a conscripted army.

result from the inability to specify or measure the outputs that are sought. If only some of the outputs are measured, however eloquent the words concerning other outputs, a budget or treasury official may tend to focus on those outputs which have numbers (economic values) attached to them. Further, because of the investment orientation of the analysis, often reflecting the investment orientation of the policy-maker, we may come to overvalue programmes that have an impact on future productivity and undervalue programmes that relieve pain, distress, concern, and suffering but have little or no impact (or measurable impact) on productivity. It may, indeed, be that programmes addressed to disabling conditions and to diseases involving mortality rather than to conditions that do not remove the person from economic activity should be favoured. That conclusion, however, should not be reached primarily because some things can be measured while others cannot. The analyst may discount the nature of the difficulty and the likelihood that this might occur, believing that his description of the items (particularly, benefits) that cannot be measured will suffice to alert the decision-maker to the inadequacy of the numbers. I suggest, however, that the analyst may underestimate the problem. He would do well to consider how compelling numbers are to finance officials and how high a rate of discount is applied to words, however well turned the phrases may be. There are those who feel that this danger is surmounted because all programmes are likely to have non-measurable by-products. They, therefore, believe that there is value in assessing the part of the iceberg that is visible (even if one cannot do the same for that part that lies below the surface of the waters). It is argued that it is, after all, better to know something than to know nothing (knowledge thus being equated with measurement and the inability to quantify equated with ignorance). Yet, there is little reason to believe that the ratio of measured to nonmeasured is the same in all programmes. If in some icebergs a higher proportion is visible than is the case in others, how do we assess which icebergs are larger in total and which are smaller? It is better to know something than to know nothing.

but we dare not minimize the danger that in knowing something we may behave as if we know everything.

In reference to quantification and its dangers, one cannot help but be impressed by the words of Charles Henry Hull who, in his introduction to *The Economic Writings of Sir William Petty*, published in 1899, noted that Petty was sometimes careless in his calculations. He indicated that Petty was aware of the conjectural character of his numbers and that Petty had written: 'I hope that no man takes what I say about the living and dyeing of men for a mathematical demonstration.' Hull continued:

> But in the ardour of argument he was himself more than once mislead into fancying that his conclusions were accurate because their form was definite. His mistake is not without its modern analogies. Mathematical presentations of industrial facts, both symbolic and graphic, have by their definiteness, encouraged many an investigator in the false conceit that he now knew what he sought, whereas he had at most but a neat name for what he sought to know. Nevertheless the substitution of symbols for Petty's 'terms of number' is an improvement in this, that calculations made in symbols must be consciously translated into the terms of actual life before any practical use—or misuse—can be made of them, whereas calculations in figures of number, weight, and measure are already concrete and appear to tell something intelligible even to a common man (24).

The danger that Hull recognized is our concern. Almost three-quarters of a century have passed since Hull, but the problem has not been solved.

The second problem that arises when we concentrate our measurement on earnings is even more basic. The previous discussion addressed itself to difficulties that can, perhaps, be solved by acquainting the decision-maker with the inadequacy of the methodology, by requiring that all analysts be humble and all decision-makers be wise (requirements that are not easy to achieve). They can be solved by recognizing that *quantification is not a substitute for judgement* but a contributor to it. The problem to which we now turn is, I believe, even more severe for it asks the basic question whether programmes are to be evaluated primarily on the basis of 'investment criteria'? Does the measurement of a person's worth in terms of his productive contribution really represent our social values?

I believe that it does not do so. In particular, it fails adequately to take account of equity and distributional considerations (which many believe to be one of the major functions of government). Note that the theory says that in instituting a programme and measuring the benefits we ask what impact the programme would have on the earning power of the individual. Because we cannot count *the* individual we tend, in our measurements, to deal with groups of individuals and with averages. Always, however, the theory would have us include as many characteristics of individuals as are relevant to the projection of future income and as are available to us: the sex and age of the people affected, their urban–rural and racial characteristics, their income and education levels, and so forth. A programme directed at women would use the average income of women as a measure of benefit. A programme directed at a specific age-group should (and does) use the discounted value of future earnings of that age-group (yielding different answers for persons in the age-group 45–55 than for persons in the age-group 25–35). Yet, taking account of the individual's characteristics (or classifying the individual as a member of a group that has certain average behaviour patterns) could lead us to direct our health activities towards those with the highest potential incomes and away from those whose earning capacity would be low: away from those with less education and skills, from the poor (whose increase in potential income may also be low), from those in low productivity sectors such as agriculture, and so forth. It would also mean that programmes directed at females would compete unfavourably with programmes for males, that the old would compete unfavourably with the young. The latter two biases are offset because income is often imputed to women since the difficulty with using an earned income test is obvious and because in the case of the young the discount rate that is applied to future earnings has a very powerful effect in reducing the present value of future earnings. None the less, the problem is clear and particularly so for the present poor since their potential increase in earnings, however large in percentage terms, may be small in absolute terms, and it is the absolute that is measured.

It is apparent that the theory and the results that would be obtained were the theory followed, stand in conflict with our value system. The victims, in many cases, of past discrimination would be discriminated against again because, as a result of past discrimination, they are 'worth less' in economic terms—and all this at a time when many feel that past discrimination justifies and necessitates compensation. In fact, the conflict does not arise because practice departs from theory. The analysis does not include all the information that it might. We are sufficiently sensitive to the problem of distributional equity that we do not include all the characteristics of the population to be affected in the projection of future income and thus in the benefit-cost calculation. In general, we ignore differences in education, in present income (at given ages), in occupation, and in other variables that might affect future earnings of different groups. The issue, therefore, is not raised because we are 'getting the wrong answers' but, rather, in order to alert us to the fact that the conceptual and philosophical problems at issue have not been adequately addressed or resolved. These may not have been problems in earlier days when the arguments presented were cast in general terms and were in support of health, education, and other general programmes. It is an issue when the analysis and arguments are addressed to problems of choice as between alternative programmes *for alternative population groups*. Often the analytical issues are viewed as technical matters relating to how economists measure value. We must recognize that measurement is more than a matter of technical procedures but that it carries with it an implicit value system and orientation. To suppose that economics is value free and that measurement is neutral is incorrect. Explicit discussion of the value system would be valuable for the debate would illuminate matters which now are buried within jargon, regression equations, and technical considerations that few decision-makers are totally familiar with. Cost-benefit analysis is too important to be left to analysts or economists. It is more than regrettable that philosophers, historians, students of intellectual thought, and others have neglected this area of inquiry.

That the calculation of benefit-cost ratios entails other difficulties is well known. Many of these difficulties bear discussion. I propose, however, to address one remaining question, not technical in nature. It relates to the impact of the kind of analysis that we are reviewing. While much of the analytical effort stems from an attempt at rational decision-making and involves a pressure to depart from incremental budget-making, I would suggest that the (benefit-cost) analytical effort is likely to result in the development of small, innovative, experimental programmes (all this is desirable) but likely to favour a 'conservative' response towards bold, new, and large departures from existing policies, programmes, and patterns of organization and funding. In my view this is undesirable. There are times when large changes are needed.

Social revolutions, bold new departures in social policy, massive changes in the prevailing patterns of health financing or organization can probably not be subjected to rigorous benefit-cost analysis. Nor is it likely that when analysis could be undertaken, it could withstand the critics of the benefit-cost ratios that might offer support for such changes and departures. At the present time we do not know how much good is created by a physician visit, what benefits more medical care brings, what the contribution of other factors is to the level of health. If policies must be justified with quantitative arguments and economic data, we are likely to find that those who would delay the institution of new programmes could argue that more experimental effort is required, that we are not quite ready, that the programme is 'good' but that it may not be the 'best'. I rather doubt Britain would have a National Health Service had the decision involved the kind of analysis I describe. This is not because the analysis would have suggested that the NHS was undesirable (though since benefit-cost analysis would likely not have taken adequate account of one of the important objectives of the programme, distributional equity, benefits would have been understated) but rather because the analysis would have revealed many 'unknowns' and would thus have favoured the point of view of those who believed in more small experiments. The analytical effort is likely to reveal that there is much we do not know and thus will favour marginal change in the *status quo* 'until we know more'. But there will always be more to know, more programmes to analyse.

I do not argue that every revolution is good (though that may often be the case with social programmes involving distributional equity). I simply argue that it is difficult to justify most revolutions on an *ex-ante* basis in the face of critics who are trying to avoid risks. In the analytical effort, after all, there is a climate of opinion which says that the programme can be justified only when we are certain that there is no other programme that is better. As I look at the social legislation enacted in the United States in recent years, I am forced to conclude that we have been well served by decision-makers who were willing to reach decisions and move on to new paths, battling for the answers given them by their ideological convictions. The programmes might, of course, have been better constructed. Not all of them have been successes, and some of them have left much to be desired. It is not clear, however, that had the analyst been listened to that the programmes would have been better. They might simply not have existed ('let's wait and do more research').

The reader will note that these comments are not based on the additional possibility that the benefit-cost ratio for a programme that is massive in scope might differ greatly from the ratio for the small experiment. If this is the case then no experiment (other than one involving the massive change) can give us the right answer. This may well be the case with social programmes that involve behavioural characteristics that are influenced by the fact that one is involved in an experiment, discontinuities, or long periods of time before their impacts can be fully assessed. The argument presented here is a more limited one, however. Here the issue is the flavour of the exercise, what

I believe, is a bias against big changes. Perhaps benefit-cost analysis has a non-incremental impact on the budget for existing programmes and an incremental impact on experimentation. One may, therefore, favour it. It should be recognized, none the less, that incremental experiments are different from programme changes, particularly major ones.

It should also be clear that I am not suggesting that all analysis is without value and that major changes in programmes should be supported by statements of faith. Our discussion relates to benefit-cost analysis, not to analysis in general. That economists (and others) can conduct useful analysis of the distributional impact of cash transfer programmes, for example, should be evident. Their efforts at constructing more equitable and more efficient transfer programmes—some of them, indeed, representing major new departures—should not go unrecognized. Our discussion is not meant to detract from this type of analytical work. The ability to provide economic analysis of programmes where the objective is simply distributional does not mean that there exists an equal ability to provide analysis of the ultimate benefits of programmes whose aim is not solely distributional or whose aim involves levels of performance via redistribution of services rather than money.

It is also useful to note one specific contribution to decision-making that can be derived from cost-effectiveness analysis, a mode of analysis close to, but not identical with, cost-benefit analysis. Let us assume that, in one way or another—perhaps through the political process responsive to and leading the electorate—a decision is reached to accomplish a certain purpose, to achieve a goal, to reach an objective, say in health. Whether it is the most worthwhile purpose, goal, or objective in terms of maximizing total satisfaction is no longer the issue. The particular output sought can usually be achieved in a variety of different ways, that is, with different combinations of resource inputs. In cost-effectiveness analysis we seek the optimal, economically efficient combination of these inputs so that resources are not wasted and so that they might, therefore, be available for other purposes. The object is to minimize cost per unit of output (or one may put it as maximizing output per unit cost). Because of the problems engendered by multiple outputs, each with different values and, thus, requiring some comparison of the values of the outputs (of the benefits), cost-effectiveness analysis does tend, at times, to move closer and closer to benefit-cost analysis. None the less, the purpose to be served by the cost-effectiveness inquiry is different.

Cost-effectiveness analysis raises questions concerning trade-offs (of inputs if not of inputs and outputs). Though more limited than benefit-cost analysis, it is valuable and reinforces our need to know more about the production function. It reminds us to consider quality considerations. Above all else, perhaps, it forces the professional to respond to the question whether the fact that things have been done in a particular way in the past means that that is the best way to do them in the future. Such questions, of course, are questions that the professional should be asking himself all the time, but the fact is that oftentimes it is the outsider who can question tradition more readily than the practitioner. There are many rewards to be derived in a wide variety of government programmes from good cost-effectiveness analysis: rewards in the saving of resources in some instances and in accomplishing much more good for people in other instances. Cost-effectiveness analysis, to some, seems to involve less exciting issues than is the case in benefit-cost analysis. None the less, the benefit-cost ratio of this kind of work is likely to be extremely high. Major government stimulus of this kind of analysis is justified.

4. CONCLUSIONS

I have raised a number (though by no means all) of the problems that relate to the evaluation of the economic benefits of health (and other social) programmes. Yet, earlier, I indicated the need for evaluation, for the kind of thinking that is involved in the comparison of programmes, and for doing so in an explicit manner in order to improve decision-making. Where does that leave us? What contribution can the successors to Petty, Chadwick, and others make?

It should, I think, be clear that in my view we have not arrived at a stage where benefit-cost analysis can be as helpful as some (but not all) of its proponents believe to be the case in the allocation of scarce resources in public policy decisions. We are a long way (and will always remain a long way) from being able to allocate the total government budget as between competing priorities on the basis of this kind of analysis. Even more limited objectives are beyond our attainment. In the United States, major elements of the Federal budget for health, education, and welfare fall within one department, the Department of Health, Education, and Welfare. Yet, competing claims between the three major activities in that one department cannot be significantly illuminated and even partially resolved by benefit-cost analysis. Indeed, I rather doubt that, given the state of our data systems and the conceptual problems yet to be solved, the analytical effort can be more than only somewhat helpful in allocating scarce dollars within a single broad line of activity, say within the health arena. Helpful, yes, because it will force explicit statements about our ignorance, because it will help us to implement data and reporting systems, because it will provoke debate leading to questions and, in some cases, answers. The degree of usefulness will, however, depend on how wise the decision-maker is, how sceptical he is of measurement techniques even as he supports, encourages, and assists in their development.

Thus we are not called upon to declare a moratorium on this type of analysis. To do so would, in my view, be an error. That we will find fewer answers than we seek is clear, but we will learn much in the formulation of the questions and in the seeking of the answers. Economists have until recently been underrepresented in departments and agencies concerned with social programmes and all of us, I believe, have paid a price for this underrepresentation. The economist's point of view, his questions, his perspective, are useful in forcing persons to examine a problem that they are professionally familiar with from another point of view. It leads, therefore, to a more intelligent debate concerning programmes, issues, and goals. Since many of the programmes referred to are concerned with human behaviour and response, departments should also increase the number of behavioural and social scientists involved from disciplines other than economics. By focusing on the economist, I in no sense mean to ignore the potential contribution of the sociologist, anthropologist, psychologist, social psychologist, and others. My own background does permit me, however, to speak with more knowledge about the role that economic analysis and the thought process of the economist can play.

In my view the contribution of economists and analysts can be important. The scepticism that I have concerning some of the answers provided by cost-benefit analysis in no way detracts from my view about the potential contribution derived from the thought process, from the way of thinking about problems. Furthermore, Chadwick was correct when he stated that economists had a contribution to make. The contribution does not depend on the ability to measure whether removing persons from London during a plague yields a return of £84, or of £72, or of £129 per pound expended. This will not often enable us to answer whether this or some other programme is a 'better' investment. But policy-makers and others need to be reminded that there are economic returns to health programmes, that good health can be supported on investment grounds, that there are high costs (for the issue is total costs, both direct budget outlays and indirect costs associated with loss of production) as a consequence of poor health and inadequate education. Economics can help point up these issues. It can—and should—serve the protagonist (not only the decision-maker). The discipline is not debased by such analysis nor is the public decision process harmed for far too often health and education appropriations are insufficient not because other programmes yield a higher rate of return, but because it is assumed that health and education appropriations are simply money down the drain, yielding no economic benefit. In a world oriented to economic benefits, this assumption becomes a difficult obstacle to surmount. Too many economists—perhaps afraid of being accused of being part sentimentalist and moralist and because of their desire to assume the stance of 'objectivity'—have been on the defensive too long. Too often we have said that health and education are valuable but that society must choose the most valuable programme, and we cannot be certain which of the many possible activities are the most valuable. While this is true and important, we must recognize that in the political world those who would compete with health and education for funds often are far less objective and analytical. To subject health activities to analysis while, for example, leaving the military budget to emotional arguments is hardly to fight for scarce dollars on even terms. Surely I am not arguing for the end of the analytical effort, but rather for a greater willingness to do what Petty and Chadwick did: to bring supporting evidence for their point of view without that self-consciousness that some of us often have because we have not examined every alternative; to be willing to say that this is good even if we cannot yet say that this is best.

Earlier I noted that a major function of many government programmes is to achieve a more equitable distribution of goods and services. The early history of economic analysis in the health field did not rest its case for an increased effort on the part of government on these grounds nor, as has been indicated, does the present effort take due account of such considerations. Clearly, however, distributional equity does provide an important rationale for many health programmes. To that extent, the task of the analyst and of the data and reporting system is made easier. If the objective of the legislature is to equalize services, to make available to certain population groups services which they would otherwise not be able to purchase in the market, services which people believe to be important (even if, in fact, they are less important or beneficial than is imagined), then the evaluation effort is much simpler. At present, in the United States, beset as we are by divisions and by tensions, distributional considerations lie at the heart of many of our problems. The healing of social wounds (not an unimportant objective even if its benefits cannot be quantified in monetary terms) may, today, be more readily accomplished by providing the services that people believe to be important than by providing that which the analyst has tentatively determined is most beneficial. The healing of social wounds is, at this moment, I believe more vital that the healing of disease. Though there is surely a relationship between the two efforts, and they need not be in conflict, there may well be a trade-off between them. In that case, social harmony would, I suggest, be the overriding goal. It may, for example, be that certain medical procedures cannot be justified on economic grounds and, in fact, contribute very little to better health. If, however, they are available to many in the population and are utilized (even if this means that individuals are 'wasting their money'), if the population believes them to be important, society may be compelled to make them available to all. This, though in many ways a more limited objective, is not a trivial one at all. We are a long way from its attainment and would do well to pursue it with vigour and commitment.

That distributional equity in the delivery of services is a limited goal should, none the less, be clear. An enlightened society will attempt to achieve a greater equity in outcomes rather than in inputs. In the United States, in the field of education there was a time when equality meant that children should attend schools with equal inputs. Difficult as it may be to achieve such goals, the formulas required for their attainment are easy to construct and require little knowledge of the educational process. Evaluation in such a context requires simple data. Today, however, equality of educational opportunity has come to mean that we should offer opportunities such that regardless of the circumstances of the child when he enters school and the environmental problems he faces while he attends school, the child should have equal opportunity to achieve a given level of education. Thus, the resources going to schools with a high proportion of poor children should be greater than the resources going to schools with more affluent children. The problem in evaluation when we are interested in unequal resource inputs and unequal provision of services so that we might have more equal outcomes is, of course, immensely more difficult since it requires an understanding of the relationship between inputs and outputs and an understanding of the production process. Thus, an enlightened society can hardly avoid many of the analytical efforts we have discussed in this chapter. We cannot find an easy way out of the analytical difficulties.

We shall have to continue the kind of explorations begun by Petty and by others. We shall have to remember Chadwick's words. We shall, however, have to carry on this work with a certain modesty, remembering the words of Sir Arthur Newsholme: 'There remains a further problem which must at least be mentioned. Is it possible in every instance to measure by means of statistics, influence and procedures benefiting the public health or improving social welfare?' (25).

REFERENCES

1. Chadwick, E. (1862). 'Opening address as President of Section F (Economic Sciences and Statistics) of the British Association for the Advancement of Science', *Jl statist. Soc. Lond.* 25, 504, 509, 522.
2. Petty, Sir William (1690). *Political Arhithmetick*, in Hull, C. H. (1899), *The Economic Writings of Sir William Petty* (Cambridge University Press), p. 267.
3. —— (1691). *Verbum Sapienti*, in Hull, C. H., ibid., p. 109.
4. —— (n.d.). 'Magnalia Regni' in Lansdowne, Marquis of (1927), *The Petty Papers, Some Unpublished Writings of Sir William Petty, edited from the Bowood Papers* (London: Constable & Co. Ltd.), pp. 265–7, 274.
5. —— (1667). 'Of Lesening ye Plagues of London', in Hull, C. H. (1899), *The Economic Writings of Sir William Petty* (Cambridge University Press), p. 109.
6. —— (1676). 'Anatomy Lecture' in Lansdowne, Marquis of (1927), *The Petty Papers, Some Unpublished Writings of Sir William Petty, edited from the Bowood Papers* (London: Constable & Co. Ltd.), p. 176.
7. Chadwick, E. (1842). *Sanitary Report*, cited by the Right Honorable the Earl Fortescue (1877), 'Extracts from the Address of the President of Section F (Economic Sciences and Statistics) of the British Association for the Advancement of Science', *Jl statist. Soc. Lond.* 25, 558.
8. —— (1844). 'On the best modes of representing accurately, by statistical returns, the duration of life, and the pressure and progress of the causes of mortality amongst different classes of the community, and amongst the populations of different districts and countries', ibid. 7, 25, 30.
9. —— (1859). 'Results of different principles of legislation and administration in Europe; of competition for the field, as compared with competition within the field, of service', ibid. 22, 405.
10. Shattuck, L. (1850). *Report of the Sanitary Commission of Massachusetts*, Facsimile Edition, 1948 (Cambridge: Harvard University Press), pp. 254, 257, 258–60.

11. ROGERS, THE REVD J. E. T. (1865). 'On the statistical and fiscal definitions of the word "income" ', *Jl statist. Soc. Lond.* 28, 243.

12. FARR, W. (1853). 'The income and property tax', ibid. 16, 1–44.

13. —— (1885). *Vital Statistics*, ed. Humphreys, N. A. (London: Offices of the Sanitary Institute), pp. 313, 314.

14. CALKINS, G. N. (1891). 'Some results of sanitary legislation in England since 1875', *Am. statist. Ass.* 2, 297–303.

15. BOGART, E. L. (1919). *Direct and Indirect Costs of the Great World War* (New York: Oxford University Press).

16. GIFFEN, SIR ROBERT (1900). 'Some economic aspects of the war', *Econ. J.* 10, 194–207.

17. —— (1904). *Economic Inquiries and Studies* (London: George Bell & Sons), pp. 1–74.

18. GUILLEBAUD, C. W. (1927). 'The cost of the war in Germany', *Econ. J.* 27, 270–7.

19. HAMILTON, A. (1877). 'On the recent economic progress of New Zealand', *Jl statist. Soc. Lond.* 40, 111

20. GUY, DR (1877). 'Discussion on Mr Hamilton's paper', ibid. 40, 127, 129.

21. DUBLIN, L. I., and WHITNEY, J. (1920). 'On the cost of tuberculosis', *Am. statist. Ass.* 17, 441–50.

22. MENDENHALL, W. O., and CASTLE, E. W. (1911). 'Vital and monetary losses in the United States due to typhoid fever', ibid. 12, 519–43.

23. —— (1861). 'The British and French armies, comparative statements, 1860–61', *Jl statist. Soc. Lond.* 24, 241.

24. HULL, C. H. (1899). *The Economic Writings of Sir William Petty* (Cambridge University Press), p. lxviii.

25. NEWSHOLME, SIR ARTHUR (1923). 'The measurement of progress in public health', *Economica*, 3, 201.

Discussion

The statement by a distinguished economist—we write for our own applause—does less than justice to the contribution which economists can make in the applied field. But experience in applied fields leads to scepticism concerning the precision of the quantitative results which are sometimes provided by economic analysis. The difficulties of substantiating such results are equalled only by the difficulty of refuting them, a point well illustrated by a story about General Smuts. Asked for the cost of crushing a rebellion, he leapt to his feet in Parliament with an answer precise to the pound. When his Finance Minister protested later that it would have taken the whole of his Department six months to work out the answer, Smuts replied blandly: 'How long do you think it would take the Opposition?' It was the approach used by Diderot at the Russian court, when he used algebra to support the proposition: 'Donc le Dieu exist.' It is important not to clothe systems and judgements in the garb of precise scientific data when they are really based on value systems.

One reason for scepticism about precise economic analysis is the difficulty of placing value on equity considerations which are among the major responsibilities of government. It is also difficult to value non-productive aspects of human life. With their non-philosophical approach, most economists do not take readily to the study of history, even the history of economic thought. In a sense the introductory paper argues for balance, between analysis and decision making. Statistics are not a substitute for judgement, nor is judgement a substitute for statistics.

The location and relationships of the economist working in the health field are matters of considerable importance. Successful medical care studies require a variety and mix of skills which are unlikely to be found in a single individual. In some sense research must be interdisciplinary, but this may be achieved better by professionals who are in close communication but work independently, rather than by common research projects to which all contribute.

The limitations of the work of economists in the health field derives in part from their professional perspective. In the USA the battle in economics between theoreticians and institutionalists was won by the theoreticians. As a result institutional work, institutional research, even institutional education have largely disappeared from the economic scene with the exception of two fields in which they could not be ignored. These were labour economics and public finance, where it was clearly essential to work with real data.

These trends have had their impact on economists working in the health field. Their number has increased in recent years, but in the USA is probably still below one hundred. Many were trained by the traditional methods; as good economists they learned mathematics and the uses of the computer, and approached the health field with interests and outlooks similar to those appropriate to the steel and automobile industries. They are often unaware of the special characteristics which distinguish the health industry; observing that all its problems have their parallel in other fields, they fail to recognize the uniqueness of the field which contains all the problems. The success of economists in the health field, where it has occurred, has been attributable in part to their close association with other professionals, but also to their recognition of the unusual features of the subject matter.

The difficulty of assessing the economic returns of specific programmes was referred to in the opening paper. It is important to examine total cost, both direct and indirect, and not to be misled by the amount of money passing through a budget. In the past economists were able to make an economic case for education and health, but when the same methods were applied to specific programmes the results were less successful. Programmes favoured on humanist grounds may be found to have little pay-off in economic terms, but in such cases it is often the relevance of the economic analysis rather than the programmes which should be called in question. The problems associated with cost-benefit assessment in health and welfare are so formidable that it is questionable whether any precise cost-benefit ratio can be substantiated. Indeed there may be no economic pay-off from policies which are justified on quite other grounds and the danger implicit in the economic approach is that the economist may assume a neutral stand on issues to which he could contribute. In medicine in particular there is a great deal of humanism, of the unmeasurable, of the non-economic; it is unsatisfactory, perhaps dangerous, to use the economic argument when it is considered useful, while reserving the right to ignore it at other times.

It is clearly important to attract economists to the field of medical care study. The attempt has been made in Britain but has not, on the whole, been very successful. There is advantage in bringing in economists whose professional reputations are already established, but while some may be willing to undertake short-term assessments, they are usually unwilling to commit themselves permanently to the health field. The difficulties are illustrated by the Trust's investigation of screening in medical care, in which cost-benefit assessment was considered essential to the validation of screening procedures. A good deal can be achieved through the commitment of one or a few gifted people. In the USA, for example, the field of the economics of education has advanced rapidly, largely as a result of its good fortune in attracting an eminent economist at the University of Chicago. It is no longer possible to speak of education as a field attractive only to less able economists. It is perhaps not unduly optimistic to believe that in the same way health economics will overcome its initial difficulties and attract staff whose interests and gifts are commensurate with the challenge presented by this difficult field of study.

In medical care research as a whole the Trust has found it essential to begin by identification of major problems which require attention and then to seek the means of contributing to their study. An early Oxford conference chaired by Sir George Pickering identified the subjects of casualty and out-patient studies. In both cases attempts were made to interest research workers, particularly in university departments of social medicine. In later years, highly structured seminars have been organized, based on commissioned papers and carefully selected participants. At a later stage the same people are brought together again in order to review progress. This procedure, though it has few attractions for the universities which sometimes regard it as restrictive, has in fact proved extremely useful and is probably an indispensable tool in the promotion of medical care research.

8

A CONTEMPORARY VIEW OF THE HISTORICAL INFLUENCES ON MEDICINE

HENRY MILLER

A contemporary view of the historical influences on medicine

The purpose of this essay is to review those that have preceded it, and to seek pointers to forward planning. We have been exposed to an enormous amount of scholarly information, and each of us must certainly have profited by acquiring some ideas not previously encountered.

THE CAUSE OF HEALTH

Professor McKeown's point that striking improvement in the public health long preceded the application and even the development of modern medical concepts is well taken. His thesis that the improvement in public health arose from *improved food supplies* accompanied by *voluntary limitation of population* and by *control of predators* through improved sanitary conditions is well argued. The *first* of these factors originated in the economic circumstances of the time. The *third*—sanitary reform—McKeown attributes to social rather than to professional pressures and to the appreciation of a general relationship between infection and filth without any real medical rationale. I suppose this is to a considerable extent true, and to the extent that it is true it indicates a medical profession with its sights firmly fixed on the individual patient, to whom unfortunately it could rarely offer much more than consolation, and for the most part insensitive to the concept of disease as a social phenomenon. It is, however, certain that by the time we reached the latter part of the nineteenth century the tremendous development of hygiene and public health and the prophylactic application of new knowledge in bacteriology greatly enhanced the contribution of sanitation to the further improvement in vital statistics that characterized the period. At this stage scientific technology was already making a major contribution to public health.

The first question is how far can the contribution of these three factors be extended into the measurable future? A steady increase in the small number of diseases that are marginally at any rate diseases of affluence suggests that we cannot hope for great benefits from any further increase in our food supplies. I leave aside for the moment the possible influence of changes in the quality and of possible reduction in the sophistication of foodstuffs, the pathological effects of which are not at present sufficiently substantiated to merit serious consideration.

What about the possible contribution of classical preventive medicine? Especially outside professional circles a great deal is made of the concept of positive health, and the NHS is pejoratively described as a sickness service. I will not labour my own conviction that the normal state of most people is to feel faintly tired, harrassed, and under the weather—and that my clinical observations lead me to believe that an abounding sensation of positive health usually presages either a cardiac infarction or incipient hypomania. The fact remains that the concept of positive health is as popular with some apostles of preventive medicine as with lay journalists. It postulates a state that could apparently be achieved by the careful observation of a set of rules that vary with the writer, but which are always inconvenient and uncomfortable and usually eccentric. I question the whole concept of positive health and the validity of the prescriptions claimed to ensure it. Indeed in the conditions of life in the developed countries which is our context today, I doubt whether the classical techniques of preventive medicine have as much to offer in the next half-century as they have had in the last. Most of the diseases that are easily preventable are being prevented. I exclude a few obstinate infections and possibly some other diseases including certain forms of cancer that may also be infective and hence probably preventable. But it is not easy yet to see any rational method of preventing such diseases as diabetes, atherosclerosis, and hypertension, depression, or schizophrenia which are the main scourges of the present day. On the other hand some of these conditions can be effectively *treated* and the patient endowed with a less ambitious state of health, that amounts at any rate to the absence or control of the disease. This might not satisfy the hygienist *pur sang*, but it would be enough for most clinicians.

There is another reason why I am not optimistic about the contribution of preventive medicine in the near future. It now concerns behaviour rather than circumstances, and demands a serious contribution from the patient, both as an individual and socially. Any British patient is prepared to take tablets and only a little less prepared to be subjected to a series of injections. Not many, however, are prepared either to stop smoking cigarettes, or to exert pressure to persuade the state or city to spend their money through increased rates and taxes in the cause of reducing air pollution. And in the matter of smoking the missionary zeal of the health educator is counterbalanced by the wiles of the advertiser and the tepid enthusiasm of the tax-collector.

It therefore seems to me that neither improved nutrition nor preventive medicine in the classical sense is likely to have more than a marginal impact on public health in the near future. Professor McKeown's *second* factor, population control, is in a different category. It will almost certainly prove to be essential for civilized survival. Is it not possible that in combination with the application of new genetic knowledge it might change the pattern of disease as well as improve the quality of life? I believe this may be a possibility and would merely add the comment here that it would demand changes in the social and ethical outlook of society of which there is as yet little evidence.

At present then I am putting no money on nutrition in the health stakes, I am hedging my bets on orthodox preventive medicine, and I am backing the admittedly speculative outsider *stock improvement* by *population control* out of *eugenics*.

We have so far left out of account a fourth factor which Professor McKeown ignores, perhaps correctly in relation to past history, but which I believe is now in a position to effect great changes in public health. I refer to the effects of the scientific revolution that has transformed clinical medicine within the last thirty years. Frankly I think our contributions have been short on the clinical viewpoint, and I hope my reaction is not unduly coloured by the fact that I speak as a clinician. Clinical medicine now finds for the first time that it can radically interfere with serious disease. The rapid conquest of paralytic poliomyelitis owed much to the fortunate historical circumstances that the problem was ripe for solution and that it was also the subject of a massive planned investment. In the last resort, however, it really depended on the development and application of new scientific techniques, and I think there is no doubt that a similar approach in certain well-chosen instances could also lead to the virtual elimination of some other specific diseases. Furthermore the treatment of thousands of cases of syphilis with penicillin has made a major contribution to public health. The operation of an effective integrated accident service would do the same. There are other fields in which clinical research and application today for the first time in medical history have the potential capacity directly to influence public and not only personal health.

The practitioner of public health tends to discount the clinician's contribution because it is difficult to observe the impact of his services on mortality rates. After all, even the triumphs of the artificial kidney and the renal transplant do not prevent death from chronic renal disease in the long run. In the short run, however, they can furnish survival and function to patients who would otherwise die miserably. There are many other instances where modern treatment may not even prolong life, but certainly makes it very much more effective as well as more comfortable—depressive illness, trigeminal neuralgia, and so on. It is also worth remembering that the physician was a valued member of society long before he was in a position to have any objectively measurable effect on the course of serious disease.

His function as a purveyor of comfort and relief should not be discounted, especially since he discovered the uses of laudanum.

Professor McKeown is even more pessimistic about the use of drugs in the case of psychiatric than in physical illness, but again this seems to me a false antithesis based on a simplistic and quite untenable view that such illnesses as schizophrenia are determined by environment. Serious psychiatric illness is a symptomatic manifestation of physical illness, and since it usually lacks a basis in gross structural change and is most often spontaneously reversible, it furnishes a specially favourable field for drug treatment. In this issue I stand firmly on the side of Medawar, who has proved in other instances to be a rather reliable prophet. The mentally subnormal child who eats away his lips and fingers is suffering from a specific biochemical disease and not an attack of Freudian masochism. I believe that recent history suggests psychopharmacology as the area of therapeutics most likely to yield great benefits within the next decades.

ADMINISTRATIVE CONSIDERATIONS

Professor Rosen's informative account of the historical development of the public health services furnishes a graphic account of the past but does not point very clearly to the future, and especially to two questions which excite considerable interest in Britain at the present time—*the future of the traditional public health services*, and *the nature of lay participation in administration of the medical services as a whole*. The discussion of these issues in Professor Rosen's paper suggests that they are not yet in the forefront of medical controversy in the United States, but it seems more than likely that this is only a question of time.

There can be no doubt that the public health services in Britain are in decline. Not only did they lose their hospital function with the establishment of the regional hospital boards, but they also lost many of their medical administrators. Indeed the regional boards were staffed at first predominantly by public health officers, and since this branch of the profession has never recruited more than a handful of outstanding physicians this was not a particularly auspicious start for the regional boards. The virtual disappearance of serious infectious disease has been another blow to the prestige of the public health officer, though in this instance it must be admitted that it represents a tribute to his own efforts. In Britain the rump of the public health service in a large city consists of the ambulance and home-help organizations, which though important hardly require the skills of a physician, and the school medical service, which has never enjoyed a high repute and has been characterized by the paucity of its contribution to research. Indeed its continuation is in question at a time when the health service furnishes every member of the population with a personal doctor. Opinion is divided today between those who feel it should be abandoned and those who feel it should be significantly upgraded. The latter would have possibilities, but one must doubt whether it would represent the most economic investment of limited resources.

Today the medical officers of health in Britain are a rather depressed group of men and recruitment is anything but easy. Nor are the candidates for the Diploma of Public Health any more outstanding in calibre than might be expected in this uncertain climate—especially since the Seebohm Report will remove many of his remaining powers from the medical officer of health. Those of us who favour the administration of the service by the regional hospital board or its possible successor in the form of the area health board would like to see public health functions transferred from the local authorities and administered by the regional board, which would then accept responsibility both for the control of infection and for the extension of epidemiological methods to the field of non-infectious disease—an aspect that in Britain has been largely left to amateurs and has been little exploited by those engaged in the public health service outside a few teaching centres. No doubt this organization would also be responsible for health education and propaganda—in other words for preventive medicine in its broadest sense. Under the Seebohm arrangement the social services are already being separately organized under local authority auspices. This has many disadvantages, and especially the maintenance of an illogical dichotomy between health and welfare which furnishes a perfect locus for such failures of communication as have previously characterized our tripartite system. However, this manoeuvre was undertaken with the political aim of leaving the local authorities with responsibility for some function in this field of activity, and unless there is a radical reversal of policy, which seems unlikely, it is not easy to envisage a more rational alternative in the measurable future.

This division of responsibility between local authorities and hospital boards raises the second problem that excites debate in Britain in relation to the administration of the medical services as a whole. How far should the lay supervisory body at a local operational level be drawn from the democratically elected local authorities, or alternatively established by individual appointments from the centre? The contribution of consumer opinion to the development of hospital services has been discussed by Dr Sanazaro, and is relevant to this issue. Administration of the health services by local authorities is an article of faith in the Labour Party, and is vigorously resisted by the whole of the medical profession with the possible exception of a few very effective medical officers of health who can dominate their city's or county's health committees. It is certainly democratic and representative, but since committee memberships tend to be shuffled round members of local authorities like packs of cards it carries the risk that appointments are made to health committees or even recommended to regional hospital boards (which always have a number of local authority members) in order to complete the member's hand rather than with a view to any significant contribution he is likely to make. One effect of this is that excessive power often remains in the hands of the board's officers, who are themselves largely recruited from the municipal services whether medical, financial, or administrative. But at the other end of the spectrum is the board of governors of the teaching hospital, which is entirely appointed by the minister. Since such appointments are usually made in response to local nominations the danger of this system is that the board can become an unrepresentative and self-perpetuating oligarchy. However there can be little doubt whatever that in most instances the board of governors presents a better image to the doctors whom it employs than the regional board. When an appointment is to be made to a board of governors the members look round and see where their committee falls short. It may be in financial expertise, experience of labour organization, knowledge of building procedures, or even medicine itself —and it can recommend an appropriate appointment to the minister. Part of the success of the board of governors concept depends, of course, on the fact that it operates within the hospital administered, and not at the distance that is implicit in regional organization. For this reason it is more accessible and more inclined to be guided by the clinicians who are operating the hospital service. Furthermore the subsidiary role of administration is more evident when the administrator is an immediate colleague of his senior clinicians than a *deus ex machina* fifty miles away.

There is one other point that must be made, and that is our continuing failure to make medical administration a worthwhile career. A few regional administrative medical officers are outstandingly good. Others are unimaginative and untalented. Even the Department of Health itself has not gone out into the profession with the declared intention of recruiting winners, nor are the salaries or the conditions of service offered such as to render this very feasible at the present time. However, these are very important appointments and their holders do much more to determine the future pattern of medicine in the country than even the most distinguished clinicians. Both at regional and at central level—and if our American colleagues are correct, as I believe they are—even at the level of medical director of the major hospital, a conscious effort should surely be made to seduce a few of the outstanding young men at present exclusively bewitched by medical technology to a field which has many less obvious but very real attractions. With regard to the Department itself and to the organization of medical directorships of the major hospitals, would it be too much to hope that some of our clinical professors might be persuaded to accept such responsibilities—in the former case perhaps on loan and in the latter as career posts?

THE PATTERN OF SERVICE

In looking back over our discussions these have concerned themselves to a considerable extent with a series of antitheses —care *versus* cure, prevention *versus* treatment, and of course in the British context McKeown is right to stress the antithesis of the hospital *versus* the GP and to point out that the dividing line between primary and specialized medical care is not only the most sensitive area of the health service but also the one most likely to change within the next few decades. McKeown seems to take the line that the British division of the profession into domiciliary GPs and specialists working in hospital was a regrettable historical accident rather than a natural functional development, and, of course, the very variable pattern this relationship has taken in different parts of the world could be quoted in support of his view. However in his more detailed consideration of this particular field Dr Brotherston recognizes the division as originating in well-defined historical processes. He seems to accept that these were necessary and genuine, but he too regrets the division of the profession into two branches and especially the crystallization of this pattern by the NHS. His main concern is, of course, that general practice without hospital facilities is so unattractive that something must be done in Britain if we are to retain young graduates to keep our unique family doctor service in operation, and he favours the granting of hospital facilities to outside practitioners. It is interesting that the working party of the BMA Planning Unit on Primary Medical Care did not take this view, and felt that given adequate facilities for effective operation in the community, primary medicine could be made a career sufficiently attractive to render concurrent hospital employment an unnecessary distraction, except in a few special cases.

But present scientific developments leave no real doubt that the hospital system will survive as the functional and intellectual hub of the service. Current social circumstances render the home increasingly unsuitable for the care of serious illness, and this is what medicine is really about. Furthermore, although many of us from time to time praise the outlook of the generalist it is significant that when we ourselves become ill we show a remarkable tendency to gravitate as quickly as possible to the most highly specialized doctor and the best-equipped centre. Although I hope that the Planning Unit's prediction of a happy future for the purveyor of primary medical care comes off I have some doubts. Even if the conditions of work are good, I doubt if the first-class student will suddenly start to gravitate to general practice. Even the attractions of the 'health team' of the community centre, complete with social worker and chiropodist, will find it hard to match the intellectually exciting and challenging teamwork of the major hospital. There is, of course, another possibility, though one that is rarely broached. The GP specialist is not usually a great success—but what about the specialist GP? If the specialist is properly trained I can see no reason why he should not take part in the provision of primary medical care. Many good specialists already do so. Most experienced clinicians in any field of medicine treat their own families and friends for anything not requiring specialist attention, and I can see no reason why this practice should not be extended if recruitment for specialist duties continues to be so much easier than for general practice. Wartime experience as an orderly officer in a large general hospital while otherwise engaged as a neurologist suggests that this would be one way of maintaining the specialist's contact with realities outside his own field.

It seems unlikely that the issue of the dividing line between primary and secondary medical care will be decided as a matter of policy or on rational grounds. It is more likely to decide itself on a basis of graduate recruitment. If present trends continue, why not make everybody a specialist—but also make him responsible for the primary care of a small group of the population, or for a short period of the working week? Whatever would be ideal, I would be neither surprised nor horrified if the specialist polyclinic ended as also the purveyor of primary care.

The history of hospital development is well described by Dr Sanazaro, and Professor McKeown has proposed well-known remedies for replacing chaos by a rational organization. The present position in Britain reveals its historical antecedents all too clearly, and our failure to modernize our archaic hospital service since the war is an indictment of successive health ministers and governments. I have little doubt that most of the average and below average doctors who have left Britain for North America and Australia did so for financial reasons. The main reason for emigration of the better graduates has been lack of facilities. Whether the building procedure of the Department of Health is a charade designed to postpone expenditure, or an inbuilt disorder of the Civil Service, it has stretched the gap between planning and building to an extent that virtually ensures that anything planned will be an anachronism by the time it is occupied. This situation was neatly epitomized by the minister's wife who recently opened a new hospital in the London area, and congratulated the management committee on the fact that the long delay in the maturation of their plans had the fortunate result that they were now obtaining a very much more up-to-date article: infinite delay would presumably yield infinite improvement. Until very recently the keystone of our proposed hospital service at the present time was the district general hospital of something less than 1,000 beds. Thirty years ago this would have represented a significant advance. Today it is out of date. There is, of course, a distinct place for the considerably smaller hospital, but in the major conurbation the 1,000-bed hospital cannot conceivably furnish a complete coverage even of current specialties to say nothing of those to come. If they are to be both effective and economic these specialties must give a twenty-four-hour service and they can operate effectively only in close contiguity. The popular concept of a group of equi-potential district general hospitals each one with one or two different major specialist units is ludicrous, especially at a time when urban communication presents increasing problems. All the special units need to be on the same campus, attached to the region's major general hospital and preferably next door to the medical school. In my city all the physical circumstances for such a development are present—but instead of this we are to have the nonsense of a third general hospital, built at a distance and housing, of all things, *cardiac surgery* together with geriatrics and psychiatry. The rigidity of thought and procedure at a regional as well as a departmental level prevented rational rethinking even several years before building began, and the first sod has not yet been turned that will initiate a hospital development hopelessly out of date before it is built.

Medicine and medical requirements change rapidly and unless our planning and building procedure can be accelerated and decentralized I can see no hope of catching up with our requirements even if money were made available. In retrospect the most effective institutions in which I have worked have grown not from detailed forward planning but as a result of improvization and extension. They have developed organically in relation to new functional needs. This is untidy and the results are often inconvenient. However, I am sure it is a more effective way of meeting continually changing needs than attempting the impossible exercise imposed on us by the Department of Health of predicting exact needs half-a-century ahead. If anything is clear from this meeting it is that we cannot predict medical developments over the next fifteen years. How can we in all conscience return to our hospitals and put forward plans that claim to meet the needs of fifty years ahead?

In many ways universities are less efficient institutions than hospitals, but when it comes to building and planning their greater autonomy renders them infinitely more effective. The fifteen years during which our new medical school and hospital extension have been planned and replanned has seen the virtual reconstruction of the major university around them. The reason is simple. The University Grants Committee has let us find the best architects we can and has left it to us and them to get on with the job within our budget and with a minimum of detailed control. We know we will have to live with our mistakes, but they are at any rate *our* mistakes, and not solecisms dictated by non-practising architectural bureaucrats operating from London and with a cavalier disregard of local circumstances.

Historical considerations dictate that at some stage the present patchwork process of hospital development must be halted and replaced by an arrangement more in keeping with the functional requirements of modern medicine. Until this is done a vast amount of money will continue to be wasted. We know from our experience of the creation of the Emergency Medical Service organization at the end of the 1930s that a major conventional war could transform this situation in twenty-four months. Is history right in suggesting that this is the *only* effective remedy?

THE FEAR OF TECHNOLOGY

I hope Dr Towers does not mind my re-titling his chapter in the heading above. Anatomists have only one thing in common: sooner or later they branch out from anatomy and take up medical, scientific, or defence politics, or some other fringe interest—and no wonder! Dr Towers's contribution ranges widely over fields of semantics, philology, and a highly individualistic medical philosophy. His basic theme seems to be that modern scientific technology is liable to render medicine more inhuman, more alarming, and probably less effective. My impression is that he would prefer to be sick in a cottage hospital under the care of a physician in holy orders whose practice was uncomplicated by instrumentation of any kind. But technological tests represent after all no more than an invaluable extension of physical examination. A blood urea estimation of 200 mg will identify the cause of obscure serious ill-health entirely resistant to ordinary methods of physical examination, and exactly the same applies to hundreds of more sophisticated tests. Technology *versus* humanity is yet another addition to the orgy of false antitheses we have enjoyed in these pages. The implication that the highly 'scientific' doctor is likely to be less humane than the one whose techniques are traditional is entirely contrary to my experience during a working life spent in hospitals. The most humane doctor in my own institution is the dedicated physician who runs the dialysis service, and nothing could be more technological, more exacting, or more dependent on the intravenous infusions which so horrify Dr Towers. In one way Dr Towers follows the traditional clinical approach, in that he clearly regards medicine as an entirely individual transaction between doctor and patient, a view of the situation from which clinicians are only now and rather reluctantly trying to wean themselves. However, he surely goes too far in suggesting that there is anything unethical about validating laboratory and other ancillary investigations for the benefit of the general population. I agree with his castigation of cardiac transplantation. On the other hand he gently sidesteps the enormous benefits of the renal transplant. At another stage he compares the gullibility of the pill-taker of 1970 with the quack remedies of the eighteenth century. There is, however, one slight difference. The barbiturates really do put you to sleep, the amphetamines wake you up, and the tricyclic anti-depressives really do dispel the glooms.

One must agree with him that medicine is to a striking degree dominated by a succession of fashions. At the present time everything is due to a disturbance of immune mechanisms. However, from each fashion a residue of fact remains. The introduction of operations for prolapsed intervertebral disc in the late 1930s emphasized our ignorance of the natural history of lumbago and sciatica. After the usual reaction which followed the realization that most cases of lumbago and sciatica recover anyway, we now have a reasonable idea of the uses and limitations of this valuable method of treatment and its success in relieving intense disablement in recent cases.

On one point Dr Towers scores something of a bull's-eye, and he pinpoints an error of which I must admit myself sometimes guilty—the discovery of an unexpected abnormal laboratory finding in a disease and the application of treatment the aim of which is to change the laboratory finding, in the hope that by treating this physical sign one may by good luck in some way influence the basic pathological process. On the other hand there are a number of instances where the changes in the laboratory reading are a reliable and invaluable objective guide to control of the pathophysiological process.

COST-EFFECTIVENESS

Dr Fein's contribution to our symposium gave me great pleasure, partly because of its intrinsic excellence, but mainly no doubt because he straightened out a number of problems about which I recognize myself to have been very confused.

I was convinced by his attribution of the recent vogue of the application of cost-effectiveness and similar studies to the soaring cost of education and medicine, and to the conspicuous success that has attended these techniques in the field of big business that exerts so hypnotic an influence on American thought. I was impressed also by the stress he laid on the importance of both the location and the sponsorship of such studies in the medical and academic fields. When they are financed by government, medical, and academic paranoia ensures that they are always regarded as aids to economy. It is also clearly true that even where a study of this kind does not produce much in the way of practical help or new information it has the great benefit of making us look again at our traditional practices, so many of which are irrational, and making us for the first time aware of our absolute ignorance about certain questions to which we have regarded the answers as axiomatic. The same kind of indirect benefit often results from the attempted application of computer techniques in many fields of human activity.

Dr Fein's chapter displays a pleasing modesty. In some ways the economist's predicament resembles that of the psychiatrist. Both are expected to cope with problems that positively bristle with unknown variables, and the rest of us have little patience when answers are not forthcoming. My experience may have been particular but it is my impression that most economists are more willing than many psychiatrists to admit that they have much to be modest about.

I am entirely in favour of the study of medical practice by economic and business techniques, and I think it unfortunate that no organization exists in Britain to undertake such studies in a way that would genuinely combine independence and expertise. An MRC-like body devoted to operational NHS research would fill a real need. I believe the establishment of at least one university department of medical economics could also make a considerable contribution in this field over the years. I say this while remaining fully aware of the dangers and deficiencies of such studies. There are, of course, many doctors who shy away from the whole question of discussions about the cost of life and about the order of priorities that should obtain in the apportionment of facilities for the treatment of serious illnesses. The fact remains that we make these decisions implicitly all the time. Not only do we demand a much higher standard of safety considerations for the airline passenger than for the steel erector, but we implicitly neglect the needs of patients with compound fractures to staff a dialysis unit. Cost-effectiveness and similar studies cannot *solve* these and similar problems, but they should ensure that even if we continue to do what we are doing now, we do it consciously and not unconsciously.

Dr Fein's fear that the fatal fascination of figures may concentrate attention on the few fields where they can be identified should be kept in mind. It is also important to stress as he does that quantification is no substitute for judgement. Many of the more important goals of medicine such as the relief of pain or emotional distress cannot be quantified, but may imply a greater gain in the quality of life than professional achievements reflected in morbidity and mortality tables.

I can understand the motivation that leads most of us to look with interest and even enthusiasm on studies in the economic aspects of medicine, but I am equally sure that to lay too much stress on them is dangerous. Many medical activities can do nothing but increase expense and the load on society. The treatment of serious illness at the extremes of life is bound to increase the number of handicapped survivors in society. The partially successful treatment of schizophrenia and the return of sufferers to community life from the institution is bound to lead to an increased schizophrenic fertility. A few nights ago I sat next at dinner to the designer of the Concorde's engines, who berated me soundly as a doctor for wasting public funds on an activity the measurable effects of which are almost entirely antisocial, when it could otherwise have been devoted to the fascinating branch of specialized technology which he represented—and he was not entirely flippant. In the last resort I suspect we may even have to ignore cost-effectiveness studies and frankly admit that medicine is a counter-productive extravagance the justification for which is moral rather than material.

POPULATION CONTROL

The second historical factor quoted in Professor McKeown's first chapter as a cause of health was the control of population, and although the population explosion has not yet seriously affected us in the developed world, evidence in Asia and Africa suggests that the survival of civilization depends on its control. If it is to be achieved it would seem only common sense as far as possible to keep the best of the foetuses and to eliminate those that are faulty or potentially expensive. Can this be achieved on a voluntary basis, or is the present trend bound to continue, where those who most need to practise contraception are least likely to do so? If society cannot bring itself to sterilize patients with a family history of Huntington's chorea, how realistic is it to expect an extension of such measures to less obvious situations? It may be significant that it is only in some Scandinavian countries that operations on criminals or carriers of genetic faults are regarded as socially acceptable—and that it is only a Scandinavian country that has built atom-bomb shelters for its total population and is organizing a service of dialysis and transplantation for *all* its sufferers from renal disease. I applaud Professor McKeown's cold-blooded approach to the control of population by wholesale but selective contraception and abortion. The change in social attitudes to abortion both in Britain and in New York suggests that radical changes in public opinion can occur quite quickly if circumstances are propitious. And is population control on these lines more cold-blooded than by hunger, war, pestilence, and pollution? If indeed control of our environment demands selective population control perhaps the main medical task of the next decades will be sophisticated health education?

Postscript

GORDON McLACHLAN

The general aim of the symposium was to explore the history of the development of medical care. It thus involved a mingling of the major interests of each foundation. While its course was roughly charted on a grid designed to avoid the shoals and reefs of a two-day cruise in unfamiliar waters, there was no preconceived notion of sightings or landfalls. If there was a tendency to dwell on more contemporary questions than on those of the past, this is no more than a reflection of anxieties at this point in time, when both the United Kingdom and the United States, with so much in common in heritage and aspiration, seem to be about to embark on periods of reform in their quite different systems of medical care.

It would be ludicrous to assume that such a brief, albeit concentrated, meeting could be assessed to show a profit expressed in positive conclusions, or even by a list of major problems. That personal profit was gained cannot be doubted: but it may well be in a form of reserve to be drawn upon and enjoyed later at leisure by the various participants.

Indeed there was ample confirmation of belief in the study of history, not only to produce co-ordinates tracing the course to the present, but as a refreshing voyage of discovery, giving a better perspective on change and its effect relative to time. We are apt in our impatience to telescope the experience of years and speak of revolution; but it is undeniable that medical care is conservative in its development and that the capacity for revolutionary change in this sector in the more sophisticated societies is limited. If the potentiality to effect change and development seems now to be shifting from the individual effort to the institution or group, this is no more than a reflection of the time in which we live; but it adds to the complexity of affairs and calls for a contemporary theory of management, to take cognizance of the behaviour not only of the individual but of groups and even of the subsystems which make up medical care.

As to particulars, if perversely, one starts with the final 'round-up' paper and Professor Miller's observation, casting doubt on the validity of the concept of positive health, this is only to throw into relief the strength of the classical iatrocentric origins of medical care; and (*pace* the social theorists) if kept in balance that is still no mean basis of approach to both the history and practice of medicine. The assumption of the existence of such a holy grail as 'positive' health, does need to be examined carefully now, when preventive medicine is a fashionable concept, the implications of which tend to have great influence on the shape of policies.

If we are, as Dr Sanazaro judges, in an age in which we have moved to a systems approach to the organization of medical services, it makes it all the more important to find some suitable means of determining priorities based on truths, not labyrinthic mythologies. Whether we like it or not, decisions taken centrally are now with us. It is important that they should be firmly based on as complete evidence as possible, and directed to finding the right mix of public and individual dynamism which will ensure that the optimum benefits of science, art, and humanism can be drawn upon by the mass of the people.

The 'research and development' concept has little history other than that of series depending on trial and error, but its current scale and the developing confidence in research in action would seem to ensure it may have a significant future.

As Professor Fein so clearly indicates, we are as yet (and it is possible that the complex nature of the total system needed for medical care services is such that we can never develop beyond it) at an elementary stage in cost/benefit applications to health services. At the same time it would be short-sighted not to recognize that if we truly are in a systems age, all possible management techniques must be explored, developed, and if suitable, applied. After all, history is full of spin-off benefits from actions designed for other purposes; and in the explorations involved it is probable that we should be able to get better insights into the confusions which surround medical care practice, and particularly the way in which primary care is made available, is utilized and what its future can be.

The recent moves towards the more critical appraisal of medical education, sparked off by the anxieties caused by some abuses of specialization, and the need for finding some means of treating an individual as a whole in relation to his environment, have been in response to a recognized need. It must be acknowledged that the spreading of popular education and the attendant sophistication is increasingly having its effect on the public's perception of the constituents of good medical care practice and ultimately on what is required educationally to prepare for it. If sometimes the application of technology to medicine seems to have been more enthusiastic in pursuit of scientific knowledge than in the relief of suffering of individual patients, society itself has condoned this to the extent that it accepts the belief that medical practice is a main beneficiary of the advancement of science. Yet once again as in so many things it is a question of balance, and if *primum non nocere* remains as the accepted dictum, there is still no reason why the physician should not back both horses, and be a scientific priest.

In the present state of affairs it is, of course, in the study of the institutional field that the historical perspective rouses great interest and even suggests lessons for application, if only of what to avoid. The history of public health seems to lead to the somewhat gloomy conclusion that publicly organized personal (as distinct from environmental) services have had at best a chequered record of success. Yet, as society grows more complex and the 'enabling' institutions have to organize their servants to facilitate the application of more knowledge and to make better use of precious resources, the form and effectiveness of such institutions must clearly have the highest priority in attention and support if they are not to be over-programmed creatures whose genes provide for their own doom.

Those aristocrats among health institutions, the medical school and teaching hospital, seem to have reached their present pinnacle because of the concept that they are primarily educational organizations and only secondarily have service functions. Yet everything points to the insufficiency of this for the needs of modern society. Even if they are conceived as purely educational establishments, it is hardly likely they will meet the requirements of modern medical education. It is proper to express in the context of history, piety for a Flexner who was right for his age; it may, however, be appropriate now to develop fresh principles in relation to present needs. Indeed, to muse about Flexner conjures up the need for a new authoritative Flexner abreast of the current scene and seeking to establish and illuminate the facts about the current perception and achievements of medical schools and their complementary teaching institutions in relation to requirements of continuing and postgraduate as well as undergraduate education.

In any event, it will be clear from the preceding papers that this was not just another conference. It may indeed prove to be the modest beginning of a movement towards a better understanding of problems common to all countries.